Tuberculosis

Editor

R.S. Bhatia
Consultant Chest Physician
Model Town
Ludhiana

PEEPEE
PUBLISHERS AND DISTRIBUTORS (P) LTD.

Tuberculosis

Published by
Pawaninder P. Vij

Peepee Publishers and Distributors (P) Ltd.
Head Office: 160, Shakti Vihar, Pitam Pura, Delhi-110 034 (India)

**Corporate Office: 7/31, Ansari Road, Daryaganj, Post Box-7243
New Delhi-110 002 (India)**

Ph: 65195868, 23246245, 9811156083

e-mail: peepee160@yahoo.co.in

e-mail: peepee160@rediffmail.com

e-mail: peepee160@gmail.com

www.peepeepub.com

First Edition: **2007**
Reprint: **2008**

ISBN: 81-88867-98-5

Printed at
Lordson, C-5/19, Rana Pratap Bagh, Delhi-110 007

To

My

Respected Parents

VALLABHBHAI PATEL CHEST INSTITUTE
University of Delhi, P.O. Box No. 2101
DELHI-110 007, INDIA

Dr. V.K. Vijayan
MD (Med), Ph D (Med), D Sc, FAMS
FCAI, FNCCP (I), FICC, FCCP (USA)
Director

Tel. (O) : 91-11-27666180
(R) : 91-11-27667027
Fax : 91-11-27667420
E-mails : vijayanvk@hotmail.com
vijayanvk@vpci.org.in
Website : www.vpci.org.in

Date...December 15, 2005

FOREWORD

Tuberculosis is an important public health problem in India. The problem is aggravated by the emergence of human immunodeficiency virus infection (HIV). The occurrence of Tuberculosis and HIV infections together is a serious threat to the control of tuberculosis. Though the main form of tuberculosis is pulmonary, it can affect any organ in the body. Thus, indepth knowledge of tuberculosis with regard to symptomatology, diagnosis and treatment is essential to all physicians and surgeons practising medicine especially in a country like India. In order to educate the practising physicians, there is a need to have a concise textbook on tuberculosis. Dr. R.S. Bhatia, leading Physician and Pulmonologist from Ludhiana has taken the initiative to write a multiauthor update on tuberculosis. He has dealt almost all aspects of tuberculosis including history and epidemiology, immunopathogenesis, diagnosis and management of tuberculosis in this update. An added attraction of this book is the inclusion of chapters on extrapulmonary tuberculosis and management of tuberculosis in special situations. Other important features of this book are chapters on co-infection with tuberculosis and HIV, MDR tuberculosis and Revised National TB Control Programme. All chapters are written very lucidly and are uptodate. I have no hesitation to recommend this book to Physicians and Surgeons of all specialities of Medicine. I must congratulate Dr. Bhatia who has taken the initiative to bring out such a wonderful book.

Dr. V.K. Vijayan
Director

Contributors

Abhijit Mukerjee
Institute of Pulmo. Care and Research
Kolkata

Amir M Khoja
Director, Head, Chest Medicine
Ruby Hall Clinic, Pune

BL Bhardwaj
Associate Prof.
Department of Medicine, GMC, Patiala

BS Aulakh
Andrologist and Kidney Transplant
Surgeon, DMC & H, Ludhiana

G Narendran
TRC, Chennai

JS Sekhon
Head, Medical Oncology
DMC & H, Ludhiana

Amit Dhiman
Medical Oncology, DMC&H, Ludhiana

Jai Kishan
Head Dept. of TB and Chest Diseases
GMC, Patiala

KP Singh
Sr. Endocrinologist
Fortis Hospital, Mohali

Kanchan Bhardwaj
Associate Prof.
Dept. of Pathology
Government Medical College, Patiala

Mangesh M Dande
Ruby Hall Clinic
Pune

Navjot Pal Singh Bhullar
Dept. of TB and Chest Diseases
GMC, Patiala

NK Jain
Head, Department of Chest Diseases
SMS Medical College, Jaipur

P Bhattacharya
Director, Institute of Pulmo. Care and
Research, Kolkata

RS Bhatia
Consultant Chest Physician
Advisor, Appollo Clinic and
SMC, Ludhiana

Rennis Davis
Asst. Prof, TB and Chest Diseases
KMC, Manipal

SS Arora
Director, Senior Chest Physician
Department of Pulmonology and Critical
Care
Batra Hospital, New Delhi

SK Sarkar
Head, Cardiothoracic Surgery
SMS Med College, Jaipur

Sanjeev Mehta
Consultant Chest Physician
Lilawati Hospital, Mumbai

Sandip Ghodekar
Ruby Hall Clinic
Pune

Soumya Swaminathan
Deputy Director
Head HIV/AIDS Division
TRC, Chennai

Vikas Sharma
Dept of Dermatology
IGMC, Shimla

Vijay Agarwal
Dept. of Chest Diseases, SMS Medical
College, Jaipur

Vishal Chopra
Asst. Prof.
Dept. of Chest Diseases
Government Medical College, Patiala

Preface

Multi-authored holistic approach on a subject, giving an amazing view of diversity and similarity, is the present collection. This book on tuberculosis has been dealt in depth to provide update information about this global disease. Each contributor has excelled in his presentation to do justice to the topic, thus making the book concise, comprehensive and clinically oriented. I have the privilege to edit the glorifying contributions of my worthy colleagues from all over India. The entire subject approach, if succeeds in providing academic insights and in inspiring young scientists, I shall feel satisfied to have sincerely performed my duty.

Human is to err and I take all errors to me to be corrected and improved upon, on receiving the comments and suggestions of the worthy readers.

R.S. Bhatia

Contents

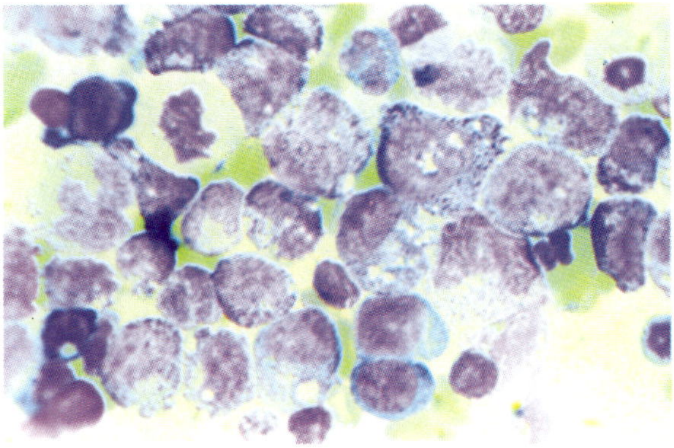

Fig. 3.1: Leukemoid reaction—marrow showing increased granulocytic precursors with toxic granulation and vacuolation. Leishman's stain × 1000

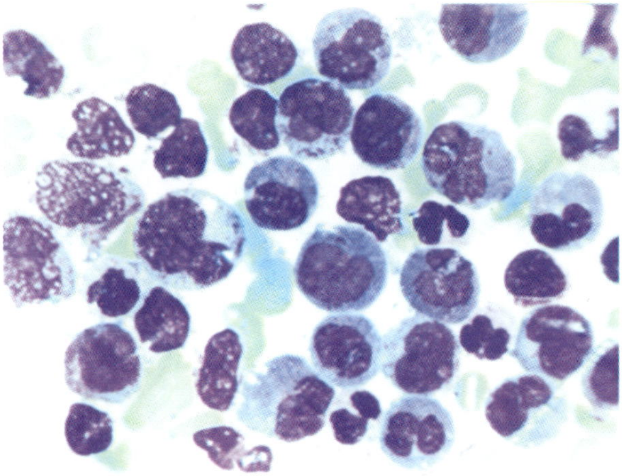

Fig. 3.2: Marrow showing increased eosinophilic series of cells (→). Leishman's stain × 1000

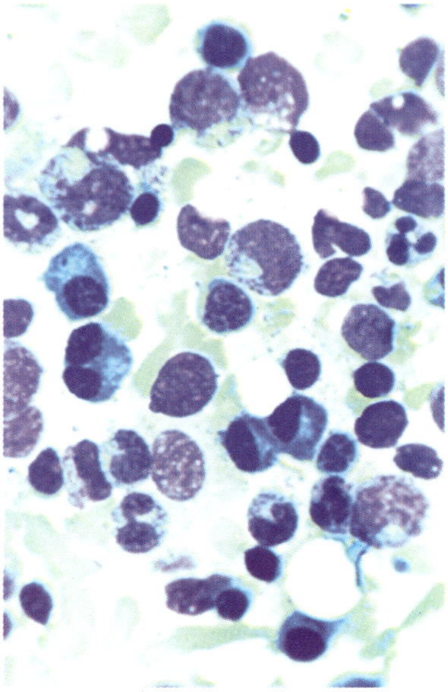

Fig. 3.3: Increased plasma cells (→) and granulocytic precursors in the marrow. Leishman's stain × 400

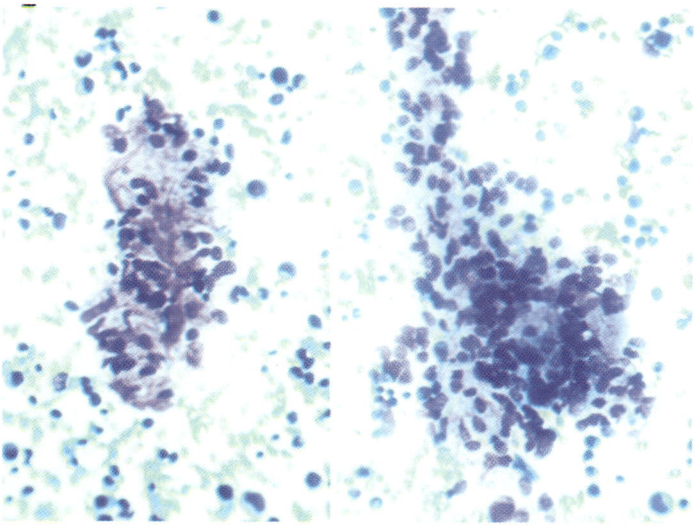

Fig. 3.4: Marrow showing epithelioid cell granulomas. Leishman's stain × 100

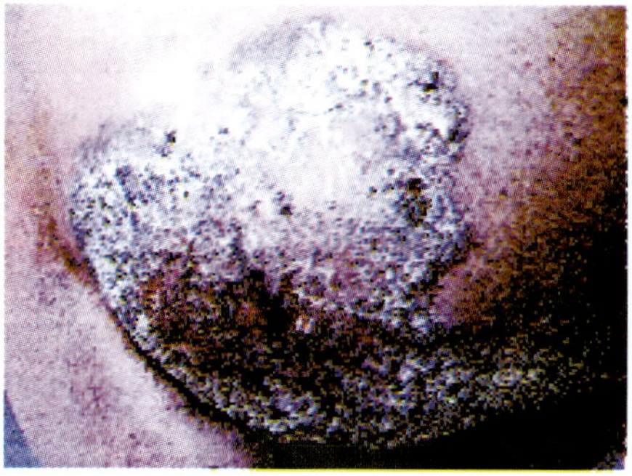

Fig. 6.1: Large plaque of tuberculosis verrucosa cutis

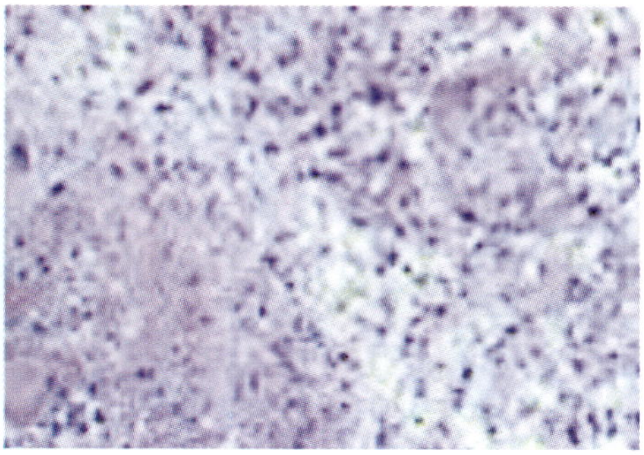

Fig. 6.2: Histopathology of TBVC showing well-ill defined tuberculoid granulomas surrounded by lymphocytes

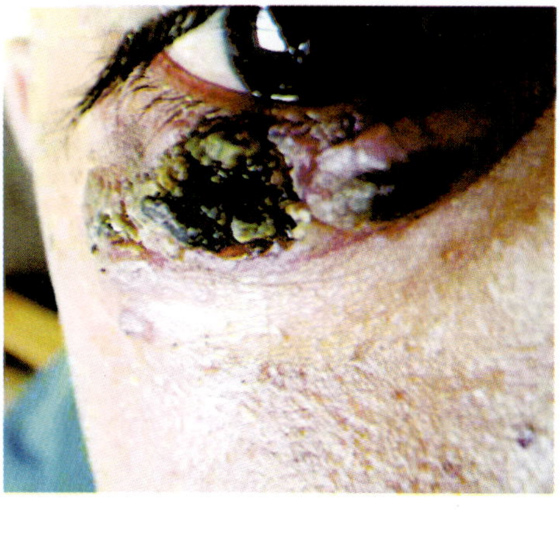

Fig. 6.3: Plaque lesion of lupus vulgaris showing central ulceration

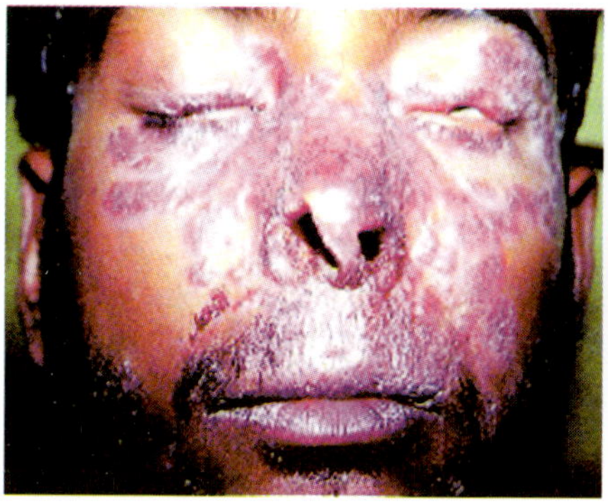

Fig. 6.4: Multiple, multicentric, papulo-nodulo-plaque lesions of lupus vulgaris distributed over– cheeks, malar area, nose, upper lip. Loss of both alae nasi, more so of left one can be noticed. Contractures of right upper eyelid with cicatricial ectropion are seen.

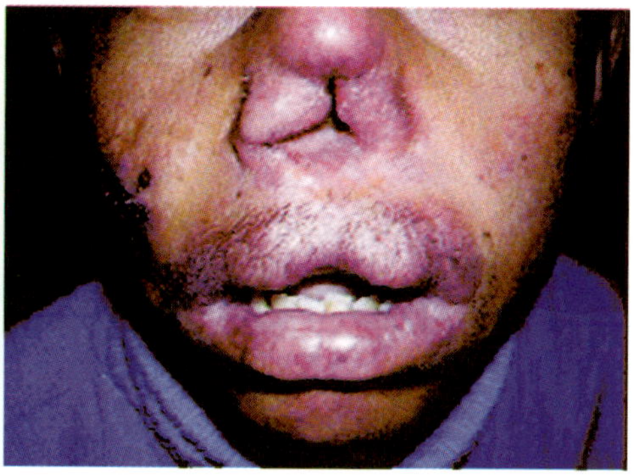

Fig. 6.5: Nodulo-plaque lesions of lupus vulgaris over nose and upper lip. Loss of both alae nasi can be seen, exposing posterior part of nasal septum. Upper lip is swollen and fissured

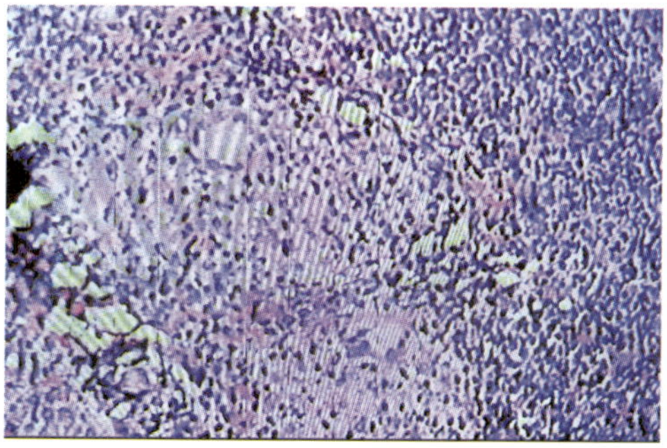

Fig. 6.6: Histopathology of lupus vulgaris. Epithelioid cell tubercles surrounded by dense lymphocytic infiltration but without caseation. There are some giant cells of the Langhans type

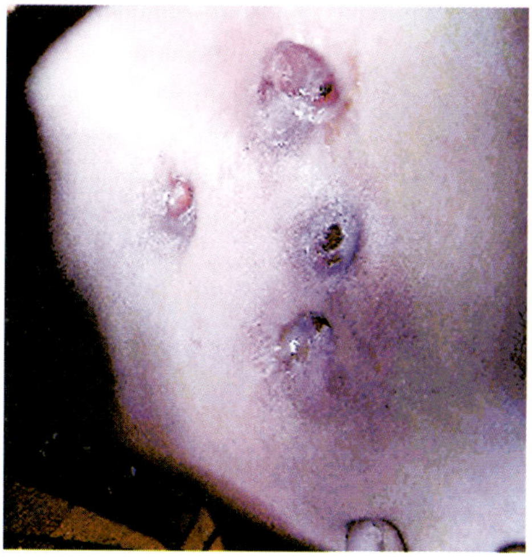

Fig. 6.7: Lesions of scrofuloderma

Chapter one

History, Epidemiology and Symptomatology

Sanjeev Mehta

TUBERCULOSIS

Tuberculosis (TB) is a chronic infection caused by Mycobacterium tuberculosis. Infection commonly involves the lungs (Pulmonary TB), though almost any organ can be affected e.g. bones and joints, abdomen, brain genitourinary system etc. (Extra-pulmonary TB). Tuberculosis is an important health problem and proper drug therapy is important not only in the treatment, but also in prevention of this infection.

History

Tuberculosis is an ancient disease. Tuberculosis was present in Egypt from early dynastic times, perhaps as early as 3700 BC. It was well recognized by the time of Hippocrates (c. 460-377 BC) who gave an excellent clinical description of the disease. In India, the medical luminary Susrut (c. 500 AD) mentioned the disease in his writings. It was Robert Koch's report of the isolation of M. tuberculosis in 1882, before the Berlin phthisiological society which convinced communicable nature of disease. Acid fast stain by Paul Ehrlich, and X-ray by Roentgen in 1885, made possible accurate diagnosis of this disease.[1]

INFECTION AND TRANSMISSION

Tuberculosis is a contagious disease. Like the common cold, it spreads through the air. Only people who are sick with TB in their lungs are infectious. When infectious people cough, sneeze, talk or spit, they propel TB germs, known as bacilli, into the air. A person needs only to inhale a small number of these to be infected.

Left untreated, each person with active TB disease will infect on average between 10 and 15 people every year. But people infected with TB bacilli will not necessarily become sick with the disease. The immune system "walls off" the TB bacilli which, protected by a thick waxy coat, can lie dormant for years. When someone's immune system is weakened, the chances of becoming sick are greater.

- Someone in the world is newly infected with TB bacilli every second.
- Overall, one third of the world's population is currently infected with the TB bacillus.
- 5-10% of people who are infected with TB bacilli (but who are not infected with HIV) become sick or infectious at some time during their life.

EPIDEMIOLOGY

Global Burden of Disease[2]

Nearly one-third of the global population, i.e. two billion people, is infected with Mycobacterium tuberculosis and at risk of developing the disease. More than eight million people develop active tuberculosis (TB) every year, and about two million die.

The table below (Table 1.1) shows the estimated TB incidence (the number of new cases arising each year) and mortality in each of the WHO regions. The incidence of all forms of TB, the incidence of infectious (smear-positive) cases, and mortality are shown both as the total number of cases and as the rate per 100, 000 population.

The largest number of cases occurs in the South-East Asia Region, which accounts for 33% of incident cases globally. However, the estimated incidence per capita in sub-Saharan Africa is nearly twice that the South-East Asia, at 350 cases per 100,000 population.

It is estimated that 1.75 million deaths resulted from TB in 2003. As with cases of disease, the highest number of estimated deaths is in the South-East Asia Region, but the highest mortality per capita is in the African Region, where HIV has led to rapid increases in the incidence of TB and increases the likelihood of dying from TB.

Table 1.1: Reported and estimated number of tuberculosis cases (and rate per 100,000 population) by WHO region for the year 2003

WHO Region	*Total number of cases estimated by WHO*	
	Number (thousands)	*Rate/100,000*
Africa	2372	345
Americas	370	43
Eastern Mediterranean	634	122
Europe	439	50
South-East Asia	3062	190
Western Pacific	1933	112
Total	**8810**	**140**

Indian Perspective

Tuberculosis continues to be a major health problem in India. TB kills more adults in India than any other infectious disease. More than 1000 people a day (one every minute) die of TB in our country. In 1997, there were estimated 4.8 million prevalent cases of TB and of these 2.2 million were smear-positive. The new cases of TB totalled an estimated 1.8 million, including 0.8 million cases of smear-positive pulmonary TB. An estimated 0.4 million people died of TB and the Indian case fatality rate was 24%. The prevalence of infection in the population was estimated to be 44%.[3] According to the latest WHO report (2005) the number of new smear-positive cases has increased dramatically[4] (Table 1.2).

Table 1.2: Country data for India: New smear-positive cases

Number of cases		*Rate (per 100,000 population)*	
1997	2003	1997	2003
274877	433271	28	41

In terms of incidence, considerable variability has been reported in incidence of TB from different regions. Generally it ranges from 60-383 per 100,000 per year.[5]

CLINICAL PRESENTATION[6]

General Symptoms

Vague, nonspecific symptoms are common in individuals with TB. Various patterns of presentation are seen, from insidious onset with mild constitutional symptoms of anorexia, weight loss, fatigue, and low-grade temperature to acute onset with fever, night sweats, and productive cough.

Cough with Sputum

Cough is one of the earliest symptoms. Initially, it may be nonproductive. As tissue necrosis occurs, sputum is produced. Cough may be mild and occur only in morning, because secretions accumulate during the night and are expectorated when the person arises. As the disease progresses cough becomes deeper and more continuous throughout the day and at night.

Dyspnea

Dyspnea is a late symptom and signifies extensive parenchymal involvement.

Fever

Although fever usually accompanies TB, as many as 50 percent of patients may fall to present with this finding initially. Fever often does not appear until the disease process is more extensive and largely exudative. Thus, febrile patients are more often symptomatic and have a higher incidence of cavitation and AFB organisms on sputum smears.

Other constitutional symptoms such as weight loss and anorexia are found in advanced disease.

Extrapulmonary physical findings may be present, especially when TB involves the lymph nodes, liver, spleen or joints.

REFERENCES

1. Tuberculosis—Back to the future, Ed: John DH, Porter/Keith PWJ, Mc Adam: 14-15.
2. TB fact sheet. *www.who.int/mediacentre/factsheets/fs104/en/*
3. Dye C. JAMA 1999;282:677-86.
4. *www.who.int/tb/publications/global report/*
5. Goyal SS. Ind Tuber 1978;25:77-82.
6. Gray SM. Pulmonary. In: Tuberculosis. Rom WN, Garay S (eds). Little Brown and Company, USA, 1996:373-412.

Chapter two

Immunopathology of Tuberculosis

Vishal Chopra, RS Bhatia

Tuberculosis remains the single largest infectious disease causing high mortality in human being. The response of the host to this bacilli is because of the interactions to various constituents of the wall of the bacillus which act as foreign substances. The cell mediated immunity (CMI) and delayed type hypersensitivity (DTH) both are involved in the host response to tubercle bacilli.

Pathogenesis of TB

TB bacilli enters the body through the respiratory route from where it further spreads to the body. This bacilli has predilection for the lung tissue probably due to rich oxygen supply.

The alveolar macrophages are the first line of defense as these phagocytose the bacilli when it enters the lungs. The bacilli is usually killed by the macrophages but if not killed the bacilli multiply within the macrophages and kill them. In stage 2 the bacilli grow within the macrophages that arrive through the blood stream. In stage 3 the multiplication of the bacilli is inhibited by the immune system i.e. DTH and CMI. The CMI activated the macrophages which result in formation of epitheloid cells and also helps in immune response mediated destruction of mycobacterium. The DTH leads to caseation necrosis which destroys the tissue and is unfavourable for bacterial growth and multiplication. In stage 4 the bacilli evades these mechanisms and liquefaction leads to cavity formation, dissemination and multiplication of bacilli.[1,2]

The tubercle bacilli bind to the macrophages by various receptors like complement receptors, mannose receptors and others.[3] These bacilli undergo phagolysosome fusion and degraded by hydrolases upon phagolysosome fusion which is an important antimicrobial mechanism.[4] The bacilli secrete certain factors which are thought to be responsible for inhibition of phagolysome fusion like ammonia.

Generation of reactive oxygen intermediates. Reactive nitrogen intermediate have been implicated as the defense of macrophages against the bacilli but their role has not been proved in humans.

IFN-γ and TNF-α mediated antimycobacterial effects have also been reported as a potential mechanism for inhibition or killing of bacteria.

Another mechanism which has been described is apoptosis or programmed cell death. This has been shown to have resulted in reduced viability of mycobacteria.[5]

But the bacilli is naturally equipped with many immune invasion strategies such as superoxide dismutase, catalase,[6] sulphotides, LAM, Phenolic glycolipid1.[7,8] It has been shown that M. tuberculosis infected macrophages, appear to be diminished in their ability to present antigen to CD_4^+ T cells which lead to persistent infection.[9] The production of cytokines like TGFβ, IL-10, IL-6 lead to defective T. cell proliferation and formation.[10,11] It has also been reported that virulent mycobacteria have been able to escape from fused phagosomes and multiply.

Immunologic Response to the Host

The response of the individual to tubercle bacilli in those who are exposed for the first time is different from those individuals who have been previously exposed.

The initial response when a person encounters the bacilli for the first time is known as innate immunity which is the first line of defense. The phagocytosis and subsequent secretion of cytokines such as IL-1, IL-6, IL-8 and TNFα are the processes initiated in the absence of prior exposure to the antigen. This is mediated through the alveolar macrophages ultimately. The various components of the innate immunity are natural resistance associated protein (NRAP), neutrophils, natural killed cells etc. The initial response is not able to kill the bacilli as respiratory burst which is required to produce toxic metabolites is not produced.[12]

Later on the adaptive response, comes into play once the immune system has been activated.

B cells and T cells come to play their part. This is body's second line of defense. The B cells differentiate into plasma cells and secrete specific antibodies. T cells differentiate into CD4 and CD8 T cells, which are known as helper T cells (Th cells) and cytotoxic T cells (Ta cells) respectively. Activated CD8 and T cells secrete IFNγ, TNFα and TNFβ. TD4 T cells differentiate into Th1 and Th cells. Th1 cells secrete IFNγ, TNFα and TNFβ and play a protective role in intracellular infections and coordinate CMI.

TH-α cells secrete IL-4, IL-5, IL-10 and coordinate humeral immunity. The inflammatory response triggered by antigens specific Th1 cells is called a DTH reaction. Recent reports suggest that the strength of Th1 response is directly related to the manifestation of the disease.[13]

The larger molecular weight antigens like mycolic acid and LDM activate the third line of defense in the form of T cell dependent and T cell independent responses. The T cells dependent response results in production of TNFα, IL4 or IL5 out of which IL4 is necessary of DTH response. T cell independent response results in production of IFN-γ and antibodies of IgM class and GM-CSF. This response is mainly through NK cells and B cells. The IgM antibody is later on changed over to IgG response.

Thus various cells and cytokines come to play a role in defense of the body against mycobacteria. The cells which are involved are neutrophils, natural killer cells, T cells such as CD4 T cells, γ/8 T cells. The cytokines which play a role are IL-1, IL-2, IL-4, IL-6, IL-10, IL-12, TGF β, TNF α, IFNγ. Out of these IFNγ and IL-12 are most important for defense against mycobacteria. IL-2 is important for the T cell proliferation.

REFERENCES

1. Lurie MB. Resistance to tuberculosis: Experimental studies in nature and acquired defensive mechanisms. Cambridge: Harvard University Press; 1964.
2. Dannenberg AM Jr.: Delayed type hypersensitivity and cell mediated immunity in the pathogenesis of tuberculosis. Immunol Today 1991;12:223-33.
3. Schlesinger LS. Role of mononuclear phagocytes in M. tuberculosis pathogenesis. J Invest Med 1996;44:312-23.
4. Molloy A, Laochumroonvorapong P, Kaplan G. Apoptosis, but not necrosis of infected monocytes in coupled with killing of intracellular bacillus. Calmette Gurien J Exp Med 1994;180:1499-1509.
5. Anderson P, Askgaard D, L Jungquist G, Bennedsen J, Heron I. Proteins released from mycobacterium tuberculosis during growth. Infect Immun 1991;59:1905-10.
6. Chan J, Fujiwara T, Brennan P, Mc Neil M, Turco SJ, Sibille JC *et al.* Microbial glycolipids, possible virulence factors that scavenge oxygen radicals. Proc Natl Acad Sci USA 1989;86:2453-57.
7. Chan J, Fan D, Hunter SW, Beenwam PJ, Bloom BR. Lipoaralinomannar, a possible virulence factor involved in persistence of mycobacterium tuberculosis within macrophages. Infect Immun 1991;59:1755-61.
8. Hmama Z, Gabathulia R, Jefferies UA, desJong G. Reiner NE. Attenuation of the HLA-DR expression by mononulcear phagocytosis infected with Mycobacterium tuberculosis is related to intracellular sequestration of immature class II heterodimers. J Immunol 1998;161:4888-93.
9. Rojas RE, Balaji KN, Subramaniam A, Boom WH. Regulation of human CD4 + αβ T cell receptor positive (TCR +) and αβδ (TCR +) T cell response to mycobacterium tuberculosis by interleukin 10 and transforming growth factor B. Infect Immun 1999;67:6461-78.
10. Van Heyningen TK, Collin HL, Russell DG. Il-6 produced by macrophages infected with mycobacterium species suppressor T cell responses. J Immunol 1997;158:303-07.
11. Moriera AL, Wang J, Tsenova Barkova L, Hellmann W, Freedman VH, Kaplan G. Sequestration of mycobacterium tuberculosis in tight vacuoles in vivo in lung macrophages of mice infected by respiratory route. Infect Immun 1997;65:305-05.
12. S Datta, R Roy, SS Gill. Pathology. In SK Sharma, R Mohan Editor. Tuberculosis, New Delhi, Jaypee Brothers 2001;38-91.
13. Alamelu Raja. Immunology of Tuberculosis. Indian J Med Res 120;2004;213-232.

Chapter three

Hematological Abnormalities in Tuberculosis

Kanchan Bhardwaj

Hematological changes in tuberculosis (TB) are manifold and pose problems in differential diagnosis. Anaemia, leucopenia, thrombocytopenia, leukemoid reaction and monomyelogenous leukemia which are completely reverted to normal after antitubercular treatment.[1] Huges[2] reported two cases, thought to have myeloid leukemia but found at postmortem examination to have disseminated TB. The importance and difficulty in distinguishing between leukemia and leukemoid reaction is stressed. Classifications of possible blood changes in tuberculosis are as follows:

I. Reactive Changes in Tuberculosis Without Dissemination

1. Blood changes due to chronic bacterial infection:
   - Hypochromic, nonsideropenic anaemia.
   - Iron deficiency anaemia.
   - Relative folate deficiency (with or without anaemia).
   - Polymorphonuclear leucocytosis.
   - Neutropenia.
2. Blood changes due to anatomical site of tuberculosis:
   - Small bowel-B_{12} deficient megaloblastic anaemia.
   - Bone-leucoerythroblastic anaemia.
3. Blood changes due to associated anorexia and debility:
   - Folate deficient megaloblastic anaemia.
   - Severe iron deficient anaemia.
4. Blood changes due to toxic marrow depression:
   - Hypoplastic anaemia.

II. Reactive Changes in Disseminated (Miliary) Tuberculosis

5. Blood changes due to altered immune response:
   - Monocytosis.

- Leukemoid reactions
  - Myeloid
  - Lymphoid (very rare)
  - Monocytic
- Hypoplasia
  - Aplastic anaemia
  - Pancytopenia
  - Agranulocytosis
  - Thrombocytopenia
- Proliferation
  - Myelofibrosis with or without leucoerythroblastic anaemia
  - Polycythaemia vera
- Haemolytic anaemia.
- Dysproteinaemia.

6. Blood changes due to antitubercular chemotherapy:
   - B_{12} deficient megaloblastic anaemia (Para-amino salicylic acid) (PAS).
   - Sideroblastic anaemia (Isoniazid, Cycloserine, Pyrazinamide).
   - Pure red cell aplasia (Isoniazid).
   - Autoimmune haemolytic anaemia (Rifampicin, PAS, Isoniazid).
   - Agranulocytosis (PAS, Streptomycin, Thiacetazone).
   - Aplastic anaemia (PAS, Streptomycin).
   - Autoimmune thrombocytopenia (PAS, Rifampicin).
   - Disseminated intravascular coagulation (Isoniazid).
7. Blood dyscrasia producing opportunistic tuberculosis:
   - Lymphoproliferative diseases.
   - Myeloproliferative diseases.

Incidence of anaemia varies from 17%[3] to 72%.[4] Anaemia is more common in miliary TB than in pulmonary tuberculosis. Anaemia of chronic disease is seen in the cases of tuberculosis. RBCs are usually normocytic normochromic, however, hypochromia and microcytosis may be observed.[5]

Macrocytosis and pancytopenia has been reported occasionally in association with tuberculosis and other mycobacterial infections. Rarely anaemia resulted due to pure red cell aplasia. Severe haemolytic anaemia is observed occasionally in patients with tuberculosis. In several such cases TB was in generalized miliary stage or involved the spleen but in others it was confined to the chest.

Leukocytosis is more common than leucopenia in tuberculosis. Leukocytosis varies from 8%[4] to 55%,[6] while leucopenia varies from 2%[7] to 46.66%.[8] Neutrophilia was a significant hematological finding observed in cases of TB. Its incidence varied from 18%[9] to 69%[6] TB may give rise to leukemoid blood picture resembling myelocytic or myeloblastic leukemia, lymphocytic leukemia or monocytic leukemia. TLC may be as high as $220 \times 10^9/L$[10]. There is marked shift to left with blasts in the peripheral blood. The auer rods in the blasts, though strongly favor acute leukemia, have occasionally been reported in leukemoid reaction. Presence of toxic granules in significant number of cases favour leukemoid reaction. A high percentage of neutrophils were predictive of prognosis in the patients with pulmonary tuberculosis. The frequency of unfavorable outcome rose markedly in patients who had a pronounced shift to the left.[11] Liver and marrow biopsy is of value in detecting the tuberculosis in patients where the diagnosis is not suggested clinically.[12]

Lymphopenia rather than lymphocytosis was observed in significantly. Lymphopenia ranged from 3.8%[13] to 100%.[4] Various factors contributing to lymphopenia were described which include reaction to mycobacterial infection, poor nutrition and fever. Lymphopenia and fever occurred more frequently in patients with far advanced disease.[4] It is also described as an independent predictors of mortality and associated with an unfavorable short-term outcome in pulmonary TB.[11]

Monocytosis may be present in actively progressing TB. Monocytes may play an important role in cellular reaction to TB bacilli. The phospholipids of the organism are partially degraded within monocytes and macrophages and cause transformation of these cells to epithelioid cells. Monocyte is thus the chief cell in new tubercle formation, where there is high rate of monocyte-macrophage turnover. This activity is reflected in the blood as monocytosis and is evidence of active extension of tuberculous process.[10] Monocytosis was seen in 77% patients with tubercular involvement of the bone marrow.[14] Monocytopenia is seen in 40% cases of miliary tuberculosis[4] and 50% cases of pulmonary tuberculosis.[6]

Monocyte to lymphocyte ratio is a useful parameter. The normal ratio is 0.3 to 1 or less. In active TB the number of blood monocytes is increased to or exceed the number of lymphocytes. A ratio of 0.8 to 1 or high indicates active TB and unfavorable prognosis. When healing occurs the number of monocytes decrease and that of lymphocytes increase, resulting in normal ratio. An absolute lymphocytosis is seen in healing TB.[10]

Reactive thrombocytosis is observed in pulmonary TB,[15] though the platelet survival is shortened and the marrow shows increased numbers of small megakaryocytes, which show reduced nuclear ploidy.[1] The reported incidence of thrombocytosis varies from 8%[9] to 52%[6] while that of thrombocytopenia varies from 1%[6] to 52%.[4] Few cases of disseminated TB can present as the adult type of immune thrombocytopenia purpura.[16] Patients who had thrombocytopenia, coagulopathy and were too ill to allow an invasive diagnostic procedure like liver biopsy, a bone marrow biopsy would be appropriate and safest procedure for diagnosis of disseminated TB.[17] A rise in ESR observed during the course of disease shows progression of the disease or indicate some complications like pleural effusion.[18]

Bone Marrow Changes in Tuberculosis

Two types of bone marrow changes in tuberculosis have been observed:[1]

1. Changes in pattern of marrow cellular framework.
2. Tubercular marrow infiltration.

   These changes result in the following alterations:

   Marrow cellularity
   - Myeloid hyperplasia
   - Plasmacytosis
   - Megaloblastic hyperplasia
   - Hypoplasia/aplasia

   Histiophagocytosis
   - Erythrocytes
   - Leucocytes
   - Platelets

   Granulomas
   - Caseating
   - Non-caseating

   Marrow necrosis

   Myelofibrosis.

Cellularity

In tuberculosis normocellular marrow is commonly seen (78% cases by Dash *et al.*[1]) followed by hypercellular marrow (in 15% cases) and hypocellularity is seen in a few cases (7%).[1] Hypocellular marrow was also seen in cases of miliary tuberculosis. The hypercellular marrow reaction may be caused by superadded secondary infections during the course of the disease or due to direct irritation of the haemopoietic tissue by the metastatic tubercles. Hypocellularity or marrow depression may be well accounted for by tubercular toxaemia resulting in leucopenia and anaemia.

Myeloid Erythroid Ratio

Majority of the cases have erythroid hyperplasia (65%) followed by myeloid hyperplasia (13%) and normal M:E ratio.[1] While some reported myeloid hyperplasia in 66.6% cases followed by normal M:E ratio in 33.3%.[19] Another study showed normal M:E ratio in 58% cases followed by erythroid hyperplasia in 22% and myeloid hyperplasia in 20% cases. Concomitant anemia and superadded infections may be responsible for erythroid and myeloid hyperplasia respectively.

Marrow Differential Count

There is increase in eosinophilic precursors in the marrow but PBF did not show eosinophilia.[19] This is explained in terms of allergic reaction of the tissue to tubercular proteins. Marrow lymphopenia (lymphocytes <5%) was seen in 20% cases and lymphocytosis (lymphocytosis > 20%) was seen in 10% cases.[4]

Plasma Cells in Marrow

Plasmacytosis (plasma cells > 4%) is seen in majority of the cases varying from 11.1% to 78%.[19] It is an indirect effect of chronic inflammation.[1]

Marrow Megakaryocytic %

In majority of the cases the megakaryocytes are normal in number (95% cases) with a rare case (only 5%) showing more than 4% megakaryocytes with thrombocytosis in the peripheral blood.[1] While a recent study showed normal count in 86% cases. Rise in megakaryocytes count was seen in 12% cases with concomitant rise in peripheral platelets. While one case showed peripheral thrombocytopenia with megakaryocytic hyperplasia with immature small forms, some of them showing vacuolated cytoplasm.[19] 1% patients with active TB had decreased platelets in the periphery with increased megakaryocytes in the marrow.[16] Normalization of the platelet counts was noted within 2-6 weeks treatment with steroids and initiation of standard ATT. Diagnosis of adult type of idiopathic thrombocytopenic purpura (ITP) was made in such cases. Thrombocytopenia is thought to be due to cytotoxic IgG antibodies directed against platelets.[16]

Granulomas in Bone Marrow

Granulomas have been reported varyingly in the marrow from 4% to 100%.[1] Granulomatous involvement of bone marrow presents as anaemia, leucopenia or even as leukemoid reaction. Severely hypoplastic or aplastic bone marrow containing caseating granulomas are present in some patients. Cucin *et al.*[4] observed that anaemia, leucopenia and monocytosis when present together, the frequency of finding granulomas in the marrow was 83% in miliary tuberculosis. All patients with marrow granulomas had peripheral blood lymphopenia.[14] Peripheral blood monocytopenia had absence of giant cells in the bone marrow.[14] This association is because of deficiency of cytokines required for cell fusion. Tuberculosis granulomas usually show the presence of Langhan's giant cells and cessation necrosis in 60 to 70% cases.[20] AFB positivity is not seen by majority of the workers.[6,9] However presence of acid fast bacilli (AFB) in the granulomas is virtually diagnostic of TB.[21] Granulomas regress or disappear in 12 to 27 days after the start of ATT.[22] Failure of detecting the granulomas is because of improper history of treatment. An increased number of mast cells is also seen. Bone marrow biopsy has a value in diagnosis of disseminated infection by mycobacterium tuberculosis, when the disease is not otherwise apparent.[23] Bone biopsy rather aspiration was more likely to yield granuloma.[24] Importance of serial sectioning was stressed to confirm the diagnosis.[25,26]

Antitubercular Drug Induced Haematological Changes

Anaemia resulting from ATT may be megaloblastic, autoimmune haemolytic, sideroblastic. They result from INH, Rifampicin and Para-amino salicylic acid (PAS).[27] The sideroblastic anaemia reverses on withdrawal of the drug and pyridoxine administration. Sideroblastic anaemia occasionally occurs with pyrazinamide. INH produces an immune mediated pure red cell aplasia. Megaloblastic anaemia results from PAS induced malabsorption. Leukopenia, agranulocytosis and aplastic anaemia occurs after INH, rifampicin and PAS administration. Leukopenia is rare with ethambutol use.[28] PAS produces atypical lymphocytes simulating infectious mononucleosis. Rifampicin produces immune mediated thrombocytopenia. Antibodies of IgG and IgM are present in these patients. INH, pyrazinamide and streptomycin may produce thrombocytopenia.[28] INH therapy may result in disseminated intravascular coagulation (DIC) and acquired factor XIII deficiency due to inhibitors which are IgG antibodies.[29] There is increased incidence of deep vein thrombosis in patients taking rifampicin.[28]

Photomicrographs of Bone Marrow

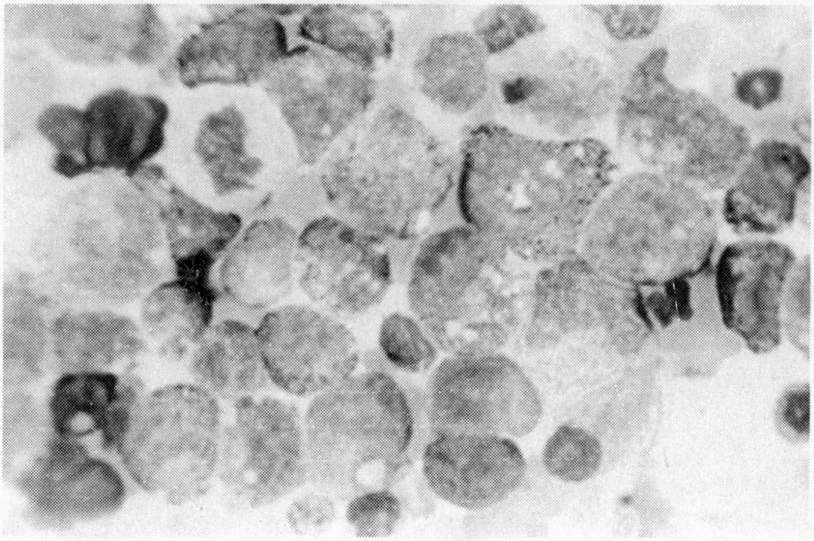

Fig. 3.1: Leukemoid reaction—marrow showing increased granulocytic precursors with toxic granulation and vacuolation. Leishman's stain × 1000 ***(See also Colour Plate 1)***

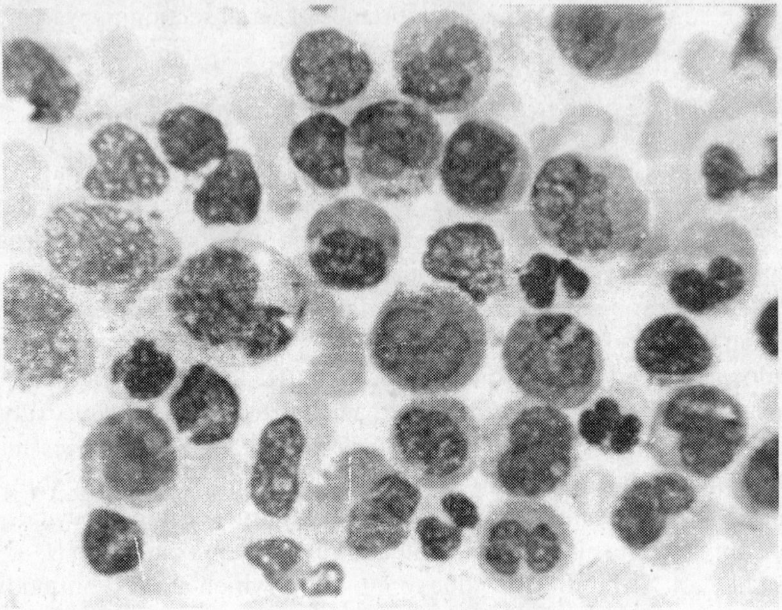

Fig. 3.2: Marrow showing increased eosinophilic series of cells (→). Leishman's stain × 1000 ***(See also Colour Plate 1)***

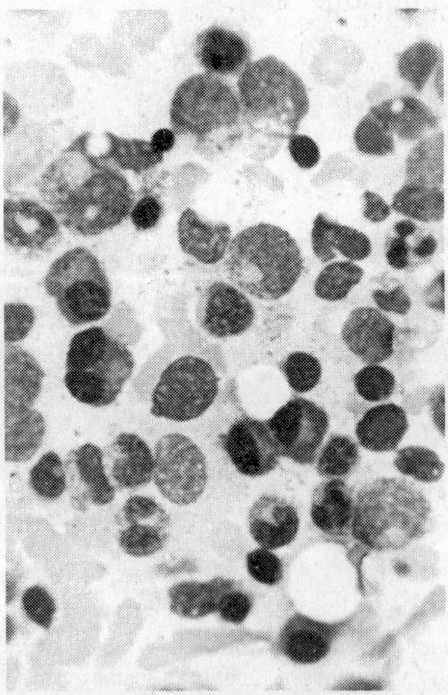

Fig. 3.3: Increased plasma cells (→) and granulocytic precursors in the marrow. Leishman's stain × 400 ***(See also Colour Plate 1)***

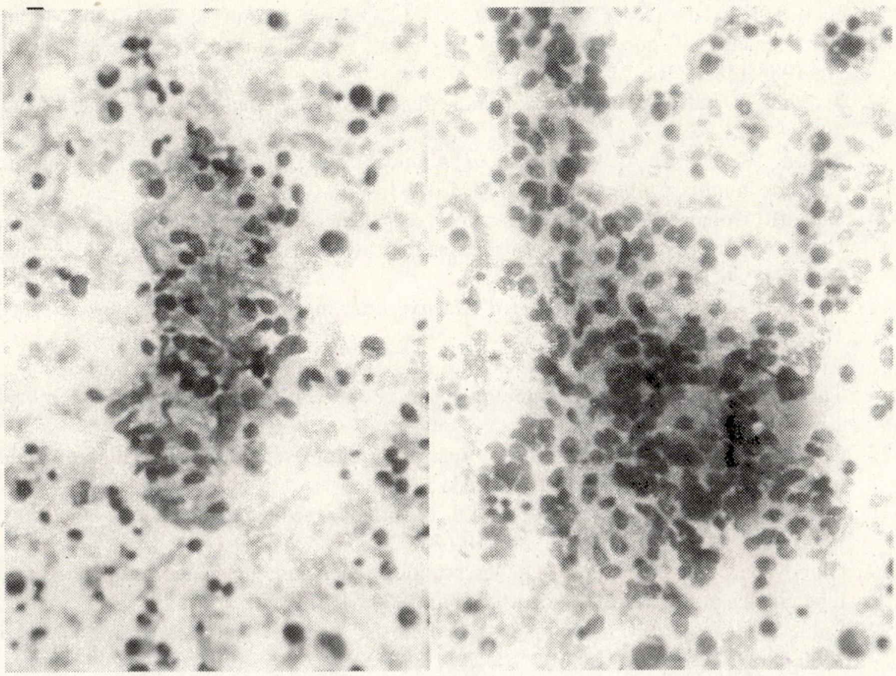

Fig. 3.4: Marrow showing epithelioid cell granulomas. Leishman's stain × 100 ***(See also Colour Plate 2)***

REFERENCES

1. Dash S, Samal KC, Nanda BK, Pardhan AC, Naik UP and Tripathy SN: Bone marrow picture in tuberculosis. Ind J Med Sci. 1971;25(3):175-79.
2. Huges JT, Johnstone RM, Scott AC and Stewart PD: Leukemoid reactions in disseminated tuberculosis. J Clin Pathol. 1959;12:307-11.
3. Corr WP, Kyle RA and Bowie EJW: Haematological changes in tuberculosis. Am J Med Sci. 1964;709-14.
4. Lombard EH and Mansvelt EPG: Haematological changes associated with miliary tuberculosis of the bone marrow. Tubercle and Lung Disease 1992;774:31-35.
5. Means RJ: The anaemias of chronic disorders. In: Lee GR, Forester J, Leukens J *et al.*, Eds. Wintrobe's Clinical Haematology. 10th Ed, Vol-2, Baltomore: Williams and Wilkins, 1999:1011-21.
6. Morris CD: The radiography, haematological and biochemistry of pulmonary tuberculosis in the aged. QJ Med 1989;71(266):529-36.
7. Morris CD, Bird AR and Nell: The haematological and biochemical changes in severe pulmonary tuberculosis. QJ Med 1989:73 (272):1151-59.
8. Yu YL, Chow WH, Humphries MJ *et al.*: Cryptic miliary tuberculosis. QJM. 1986;59:421-28.
9. Bozodky G, Ruby E, Goher I, Toth J and Mohos A: Haematological abnormalities in pulmonary tuberculosis. Orv Hetil (Hungary) 1997:138(17):1053-56.
10. Gay JC and Athens JW: Variations of leukocytes in disease. In: Lee GR, Forester J, Lukens J *et al.*, Eds. Wintrobe's Clinical Haematology. 10th Ed, Vol. 2: Baltomore: Williams and Wilkins, 1999;1836-61.

11. Barnes PF, Leedom JM, Chan LS, Wong SF, Shah J, Vachon LA, Overtruf GD and Modlin RL: Predictors of short term prognosis in patients with pulmonary tuberculosis: J Infect Dis 1988;158(2):366-71.
12. Twomey JJ and Leavell BS: Leukemoid reactions to tuberculosis. Arch Intern Med. 1965;116:21-28.
13. Sharma SK, Mohan A, Pande JN *et al.*: Clinical profile, laboratory characteristics and outcome in miliary tuberculosis. QJ Med. 1995;88:29-37.
14. Cucin R, Coleman M, Eckhardt J and Silver R: The diagnosis of miliary tuberculosis: Utility of peripheral blood abnormal, bone marrow and liver needle biopsy. J Chronic Dis. 1973;26:355-61.
15. Baynes RD, Bothwell TH, Flax H *et al.* Reactive thrombocytosis in pulmonary tuberculosis. J Clin Pathol. 1987;40:676-79.
16. Al-Maj SA, Al-Momen AK, Al-Kassimi FA, Al-Zeer A, Kambal AM and Baaqil H: Tuberculosis presented as immune thrombocytopenic purpura. Acta Haemotol 1995;94:135-38.
17. Lim KH and Chong KL: Multiple organ failure and septic shock in disseminated tuberculosis. Singapore Med J 1999;40(3):176-78.
18. Marquis D: The blood. In: Maile JB Ed. Laboratory medicine hematology. 6th ed; St. Louis: The Mosby Company 1982:350-68.
19. Oluboyede OA and Onadeko BO: Observation to haematological patterns in pulmonary tuberculosis in Nigerians J. Trop Med Hyg. 1978;81(5):91-95.
20. Prout S, Benetar SR Disseminated tuberculosis. A study of 62 cases. S Afr Med J 1980;58:835-42.
21. Maatens G, Willcox PA, Benatar SR. Miliary tuberculosis. Rapid diagnosis, hematologic abnormalities and outcome in 109 treated adults. Am J Med 1990;89:291-96.
22. Heinle EW, Jensen WN and Westerman MP: Diagnostic usefulness of marrow biopsy in disseminated tuberculosis. Am Rev Resir Dis. 1965;91:701-05.
23. Watts I: The bone marrow. In: Maile JB Ed. Laboratory medicine hematology. 6th Ed; St. Louis: The Mosby Company 1982;211-349.
24. Alvarez S and Mc Cabe WR: Extrapulmonary tuberculosis revisited: A review of experience at Boston city and other hospitals. Medicine (Baltimore) 1984;63;25-55.
25. Kinoshita M, Ichikawa Y, Koga H, Sumita and Oizumi K: Re-evaluation of bone marrow aspiration in the diagnosis of miliary tuberculosis. Chest 1994;106:690-92.
26. Nakajima M, Niki Y Manabe T and Matasushima T: Detection of lesions in marrow for the diagnosis of miliary tuberculosis: Reliability of bone marrow aspiration and biopsy in view of distribution pattern of lesions in autopsy cases. Kansenshogaku Zasshi. 1996;70(9):963-69.
27. Bottomley SS, Sideroblastic anaemia. In: Jacobs A, Worwooda MZ, editors. Iron biochemistry and medicine. Vol. 2, London: Academic press; 1980;363-92.
28. Holdiness MR, Blood dyscrasias induced by antituberculosis drugs. Tubercle 1987;68:301-09.
29. Stuart JJ, Roberts AR. Isoniazid and disseminated intravascular coagulation. Ann Intern Med 1976;84:490-91.

Chapter four

Tuberculosis and the Endocrine System (Metabolic Changes in TB)

KP Singh

Mycobacterium tuberculosis has been described to infect virtually every endocrine gland help; however the incidence of endocrine gland involvement is low, especially in the era of effective anti mycobacterial chemotherapy. Furthermore, the administration of anti-tuberculosis drugs has been associated with endocrine effects.

Adrenal Gland

Worldwide, infections are the most common cause of adrenal insufficiency that comprise tuberculosis, fungal infection and cytomegalovirus infection. Tuberculosis may affect many of the endocrine glands including the hypothalamus, pituitary, thyroid and adrenals. The most commonly involved endocrine organ in tuberculosis is the adrenal gland. Adrenal glands may be directly or indirectly affected by tuberculosis. Tuberculosis Addison's disease is still an important cause of primary adrenocortical insufficiency particularly in the developing countries. Recent improvements in imaging techniques and modern endocrinological tests for the investigation of adrenal function have given us greater insight into the endocrinology of adrenal tuberculosis.

Hypothalamo-pituitary-adrenal (HPA) axis is also involved in tuberculosis and recent findings revealed that HPA axis is activated rather than under-activated in active pulmonary tuberculosis. Activated HPA axis is tuberculosis causes increased cortisol secretion which results in a shift in the Th1/Th2 balance towards Th2, T cell dysfunction due to high cortisol and low DHEAS levels may be responsible for immunologically-mediated tissue damage in tuberculosis.

The histological findings of adrenal tuberculosis shows four patterns, caseating or noncaseating granulomas, glandular enlargement with adrenal destruction by inflammatory granulomas, mass lesions secondary to the development of cold abscesses, and adrenal atrophy from fibrosis related to chronic infection. Calcification of the gland is a common but not specific finding. The adrenals are initially enlarged with extensive epithelioid granulomas and caseation and both the cortex and the medulla are affected. Fibrosis ensues and the adrenals become normal or smaller in size with calcification evident in 50% cases.

Tuberculous Addison's disease results from haematogenous spread of infection from elsewhere in body and extradrenal disease is usually evident. Sign and symptoms of insufficiency appear when approximately more than 90% of the gland is destroyed. Treatment recommendations for adrenal tuberculosis are similar to those outlined for pulmonary tuberculosis in all cases, except for children with miliary tuberculosis for whom prolonged treatment in excess of the standard six-month regime is indicated. Suspicion of acute adrenal crisis demands immediate therapy that should not be delayed for results of diagnostic studies. There is no contraindication to continuing steroids administration patients with active tuberculosis who require steroid therapy for other indications including select manifestations of tuberculosis, as long as these patients are undergoing anti tuberculous chemotherapy.

Pituitary Gland

Pituitary gland tuberculosis is an extremely rare occurring in less than 1% of persons with tuberculosis. In a selected group of pituitary gland involvement was seen in 4% of patients with late, generalized tuberculosis.

Tuberculosis may spread haematogenously or by direct extension from the sphenoidal sinus, brain, or meningitis.

Any portion of the pituitary (including anterior, posterior, and the stalk) or the hypothalamus can be involved; consequently, presentations can vary and have included growth retardations, hypogonadism, galactorrhea-amenorrhea related to excess prolactin secretion, diabetes insipidus, and even panhypopituitarism.

Hyponatremia and the Syndrome of Inappropriate Antidiuretic Hormone Secretion

The presence of a substance with antidiuretic hormone-like properties similar or identical to arginine vasopressin from tuberculosis lung tissue of a patient with hyponatremia, which suggested that this tissue either produces or less likely, absorbs inappropriately released hormone from the posterior pituitary. Tuberculosis meningitis was reported to be associated with SIADH in a patient who had active pulmonary disease. The degree of hyponatremia is generally highly variable in patients with tuberculosis, and most patients are asymptomatic.

The vast majority of patients experience correction of their hyponatremia response to treatment of their tuberculosis.

Thyroid Gland

Mycobacterium may spread to the thyroid gland hematogenously or from an adjacent focus such as cervical or mediastinal adenitis. The presentation may be that of a nodule, mass, thyroiditis, or acute or cold abscess. Symptoms from pressure effects include dysphagia, dyspnea and dysphonia.

Tuberculosis rarely involves the thyroid gland. In a series of selected patients with late generalized tuberculosis occurring in pre and post antibiotic eras, 14% of patients had evidence of thyroid seeding.

Thyroid function test results are usually normal in patients with tuberculous thyroiditis, but thyrotoxicosis as well as myxedema have been reported.

Fine-needle aspiration for cytology and microbiology is the preferred diagnostic tool for the differentiation of tuberculous thyroiditis from carcinoma and other granulomatous entities.

Thyroid abnormalities may be noted in patients with acute tuberculosis who do not have associated infection of the thyroid gland. In patients who are hospitalized with tuberculosis, the incidence of euthyroid sick syndrome has been substantial ranging from 63-92%.

Anti-tuberculous therapy may also have some effect on thyroid appearance and function. An association between the administration of PAS (Para Amino Salicylic acid) and the development of goiters. In addition rifampin induction of hepatic microsomal enzymes may enhance the extra thyroidal metabolism of thyroid hormones, specifically decreasing levels of serum free T_a and possibly T_4 and reverse T_3.

Diabetes Mellitus

Patients with diabetes mellitus appear to be at increased risk for the development of tuberculosis. Immunologic studies in diabetic patients suggest that some significant abnormalities may predispose them to chronic pulmonary infections. In particular, patients with diabetes, especially those with hyperglycemia, have been noted to have impaired granulocyte chemotaxis, phagocytosis, bactericidal activity and super oxide production. Furthermore, monocyte macrophage function may also be impaired. Reduced number of circulating peripheral monocytes, decreased phagocytosis, and alterations in surface receptor may all contribute to enhanced diabetic susceptibility to infections with intracellular pathogens.

Insulin deficiency results in impairment of both leukocyte and lymphocyte mediated response to infection. These immunodeficiencies improve with antidiabetic treatment. The advent of effective anti tuberculous and antidiabetic treatment led to a decrease in the death rate from tuberculosis with diabetes from 5.5-3%.

It has been reported that the presentation of tuberculosis in patients with diabetes is different from that in patients without diabetes. In one study of 36 patients with diabetes and tuberculosis, there was a significant increase in cavitary and sputum positive disease. In another study, an increase in lower lobe disease was suggested.

Increased susceptibility of patients with diabetes mellitus to tuberculosis could be due to neutrophilic dysfunction and impaired cytokines production. Interferon alpha-production capacity of white blood culture has been found to be reduced in patients with diabetes mellitus as well as tuberculosis patients. Significantly lowered production interlukin-1B (IL-1 beta) and tumor necrosis factor-Alpha (TNF-alpha) by the peripheral blood monocyte in patients with tuberculosis and coexistent diabetes mellitus compared to patients with tuberculosis and no diabetes mellitus. The production of IL-1 beta and TNF-alpha was significantly lower in patients with poor glycemic control. Increased susceptibility to tuberculosis could also be due to thickened alveolar epithelium and pulmonary basal lamina, reduced pulmonary diffusion capacity, reduced lung volumes and elastic recoil in patients with diabetes mellitus.

Hypercalcemia

Patients with active tuberculosis usually have normal serum calcium levels; however hypercalcemia has been frequently noted and there have been limited reports of hypocalcemia in this patient population. Most cases of hypercalcemia in tuberculosis, like those associated with sarcoidosis and other granulomatous diseases, appear to be linked to abnormal Vitamin D metabolism levels of dihydroxy Vitamin D have correlated significantly with serum calcium levels in advanced pulmonary tuberculosis. Activated macrophage with enhanced activity of 1-alpha-hydroxylase enzyme causes increased levels of 1,25 $(OH)_2$ Vitamin D.

REFERENCES

1. Endocrine and metabolic aspects of tuberculosis; Emily A, Blumberg and Elias Abrutyn in tuberculosis and non tuberculous mycobacterial infection by Schlossberg 4th edition.
2. Endocrine and metabolic manifestations of tuberculosis: Joseph Lowy in Tuberculosis by William N. Rom and Stuart M. Garay, 2nd edition.
3. Endocrine Implications of Tuberculosis, R Goswami, N Kochipillai in Tuberculosis by SK Sharma and A Mohan 1st edition.

Chapter five

Extrapulmonary Tuberculosis

Soumya Swaminathan, G Narendran

ABSTRACT

Tuberculosis (TB) is one of the most common infections occurring in individuals with HIV/AIDS and TB rates have gone up in many parts of the world. Extrapulmonary TB assumes importance as clinical presentation may be diverse and a delay in diagnosis can prove fatal. The emphasis on clinical presentation may be so great that it leads to over diagnosis. There is ambiguity regarding duration of drug therapy and role of surgery. Short course chemotherapy regimen for 6-12 months has proved effective in obviating the need for surgery in majority of the cases. A high index of suspicion and early diagnosis and regular chemotherapy results in a favourable outcome.

INTRODUCTION

The clinical manifestation of tuberculosis can be pulmonary or extrapulmonary (outside the lungs). The highly vascular areas like lymph node, meninges, kidney, spine and growing end of bones are usually affected. In India, 10-15% of all forms of TB are extrapulmonary TB. A higher prevalence has been noted due to the interaction of HIV and TB. The clinical presentation is may be so much atypical that TB may not be considered in the differential diagnosis. Sputum for AFB and X-ray chest may not aid in the diagnosis. Extrapulmonary TB may require specialist care with diagnostic modalities that may not be widely available. Mantoux is useful, but its value is limited to children less than 5 years of age, as 40% or more of the Indian population is infected with TB. The PPD assumes importance as far as TB lymphadenitis is concerned. Attempts should be made to confirm the diagnosis by HPE or bacteriological smear/culture wherever possible. Studies conducted by TRC showed 33-62% culture positivity in different forms of extrapulmonary TB (Table 5.1). Even though a number of reports on immunologic tests like SAFA, ELISA and slide agglutination technique are available, the specificity and sensitivity are variable and need to be interpreted in the light of clinical findings. Supportive evidence from ADA of more than 9

Table 5.1: An overview of studies conducted by TRC in various extrapulmonary forms of TB

Studies	*No. of patients*	*Mx+*	*X-ray evidence*	*No. of specimens*	*Bac. proof*	*HPE proof*
TB spine	304	93	13	85	50	29
TB meningitis	180	50	55	180	33	–
TB lymphadenitis	197	81	24	168	62	98
TB abdomen	193	74	48	156	40	51
Tuberculoma brain	108	44	9	13		61

IU and lysozyme of 2 mg/litre or more could provide an indirect diagnosis in some cases like TB meningitis. Several RCT's have established the efficacy of Short Course Chemotherapy (SCC) as the main stay of management.[7] The response to intermittent regimen has been as effective as daily regimen. The International Union against TB and lung diseases and the joint tuberculosis committee of the British Thoracic Society have recommended 2HRZ7/4HR7 for all extrapulmonary forms of tuberculosis except serious forms like joint and brain TB where the duration is extended upto 12 months. The cure rate was 87-99% except in Pott's paraplegia and relapse rate was less than 4%.

TB LYMPHADENITIS

It is the most common type of TB described in hippocrates writing dating back to 460-377 B.C. It was initially thought to be cured by the touch of the king (king's evil) in Europe.

Epidemiology: Cervical region is the most common. Risk factors include younger age group, immune status, race (more in blacks). Sex: F>M. 2:1.

Pathology: It spreads from primary focus to regional draining lymph nodes. This often results in a greater volume of diseased tissue in regional lymph nodes than at the original site of infection. Further spread via lymphatic to other nodes and hematogenous spread occurs if not contained.

Bacteriology: *Mycobacterium TB* is the most common in India followed by *M. bovis* and africanum. Non-TB mycobacteria especially MAC and scrofulaceum should be kept in mind in the HIV millennium.

Clinical Features: Persons affected may have nonspecific constitutional symptoms.

Locally there may be a painless swelling with discharging sinus with or without scar. A classical presentation is multiple, matted and variable consistency of the lymph node which is painless and slow growing. Rare manifestations include chyluria, chronic abdominal pain, progressive jaundice, dysphagia and generalized lymphadenopathy.[1]

Histology: Reveals epitheloid cells, modified histiocytes, Langhan's giant cells surrounded by dense, infiltrate of lymphocytes. Caseation may or may not be present.

Investigations: Mantoux is significant especially in < 5 years of age, but may not be specific. FNAC is the easiest, safe and convenient way of proving the diagnosis followed by biopsy. CT scan of the chest/abdomen may give additional details such as mediastinal or retroperitoneal adenopathy, and can even distinguish between MTB and MAC. The presence of focal visceral lesion and low attenuation in LN suggest MTB. Marked hepatic and splenic enlargement with enlarged soft density nodes (density > muscle suggest MAC[8]).

Treatment: Medial RNTCP: CAT III with two months of HRZ/4HR in immunocompetent patients. Four drugs in the intensive phase in immunocompromised/seriously ill patients.

Surgical Indication: (1) Sinus tract removal. (2) Enlargement and softening in spite of treatment. (3) Concomitant and suspicion of malignancy. (4) Atypical mycobacteria.

TB BONE AND JOINTS

The incidence of skeletal tuberculosis is very high in children adolescents and young adults. Higher incidence of 30% occurs in young adults. It is uncommon in old age. Among TB patients 1-3% have skeletal TB.

Etiology: Like other infection, it is mostly a monoarthritis. MTB is the causative organism. It is secondary to another focus in the lung or contiguous nodes as a rule.

Pathology: There are two types of microscopic lesions. (i) The ***caseating exudative type*** with predominant necrosis and cold abscess formation. (ii) The ***proliferating type*** where the cellular proliferation predominates with minimal or no caseation. The extreme form occurs in TB granuloma of the shoulder ***"Carus sicca".***

Clinical Features: Onset is insidious with constitutional symptoms. It is succeeded by localizing symptoms and signs according to the site involved.

TB Spine: (Pott's Spine)

Tuberculosis of the spine forms 50-60% of the total incidence of skeletal tuberculosis. The most common level is the thoracolumbic region due to excessive strain of movement and weight bearing at this level. The various locations favoured are: (1) Paradisc region. (2) Central body. (3) Anterior type. (4) Appendiceal lesion. (5) Articular region. The lesion soon destroys the intervertebral disc and adjacent body of the vertebra, which collapse and obliterate the intervertebral space. Destruction of the framework results in an angular kyphosis called gibbus. Spreading caseation and osteolysis leads to a cold abscess.

Clinical Features: (1) Pain, which can be localized or referred pain. (2) Rigidity, caused by spasm of para spinal muscles demonstrated by coin test. (3) Deformity can be in the form of gibbus in thoracic region and loss of normal curvature as in cervical or lumbar region. (4) Cold abscess: The abscess forms in the para vertebral region and soon tracks downwards due to gravity and tracks down along the neurovascular bundle. In the cervical region, it forms a retropharyngeal abscess. In the thorax, it can track lateral or anterior. Thoracolumbar cold abscess can point in the back or enter the psoas sheath and track down to psoas or iliac region. (5) Paraplegia: Occurs in 10% of cases, the higher being in the thoracic spine. Early onset paraplegia occurs in the active stage of the disease. Late onset paraplegia occurs due to deformity or sequelae. A rare gradual onset of paraplegia occurs in "Spinal cord tumor syndrome", due to granulation tissue growing inside the spinal cord.

Investigations: Specific; X-ray spine: Earliest radiological sign is narrowing of intervertebral space followed by erosion, destruction and collapse of vertebral bodies with obliteration of intervertebral space.

Treatment: Anti-TB treatment for a period of 6-12 months. Once the lesion becomes quiescent, patient is given a spinal brace. Surgery is indicated. (1) When there is no sign of recovery. (2) Paraplegia getting worse in spite of treatment. (3) Spastic paraplegia. The randomized clinical trial conducted in Madras by TRC, in collaboration with BMRC, and orthopedic department of GGH in 1975-78 showed that SCC for 9 months is effective for spinal tuberculosis without paraplegia obviating the need for surgery. Surgery is indicated only in patients less than 15 years of age and having an initial angle of kyphosis > 30°.[2,3,7]

TB Hip Joint

It is the second most common site involved in the age of 5-15 years.
Stage 1: There is exudation into the joint cavity with the limb assuming flexion, abduction and external rotation. *Stage 2:* The spasm of adductors take over resulting in flexion, adduction, internal rotation. *Stage 3:* The neglected joint is destroyed resulting in real shortening of the limb.

The cold abscess opens with sinus pouring out pus.

X-ray of the Hip Joint: (1) Rarefaction of bone and joint space widening due to effusion. (2) Erosion of articular surface and narrowing of joint space. (3) Destruction of the femur with dislocation of acetabulum "travelling acetabulum". MRI and CT can reveal abnormalities in greater detail.

Treatment: SCC for 6 months, bed rest for 3 months followed by protected weight bearing.

TB Shoulder Joint: In this site, it is caries sicca of the dry type.

TB Osteomyelitis

Occurs in children, affecting the shaft of phalanges. There is subperiosteal new bone formation and thickening of the bone peculiar to TB infection of the short long bones making the fingers spindle shaped "spina ventosa".

BCG Osteomyelitis: It is a rare complication of BCG vaccine occurring in a few months to few years after BCG vaccination. The condition is benign and heals with ATT.

Poncets Osteomyelitis: It is a polyarthritis resembling rheumatoid arthritis occurring during treatment. The condition requires symptomatic management only.[3]

ABDOMINAL TUBERCULOSIS

Includes upper GI lesions, ulceration, ileocaecal, omental inflammation, mesenteric adenitis, TB peritonitis, anorectal lesion, hepatitis. Some of them are described here. (Frequency distribution is given in Table 5.2).

Table 5.2: Frequency distribution of abdominal TB

Location	*Clinical reporting percentage*
Esophageal	0.3
Stomach	2
Duodenum	0.3
Jejunum	35
Ileum	35
Ileocaecal	42
Appendix	1
Colon	12
Anorectum	7

Its prevalence increased in the era of HIV. It constitutes 5% of extrapulmonary TB in India. It can be primary from swallowing and ingestion of infected sputum or by haematogenous spread from miliary or primary pulmonary TB (silent bacilliemia).

Anatomical distribution: It can occur anywhere from mouth to anus, ileocaecal junction being the most common. The preponderance of lymphoid tissue, increased physiological stasis, increased rate of absorption, and electrolyte absorption, minimal digestive activity all favour the invasion of the TB bacilli at the site. The involvement of oesophagus, pancreas and appendix are common in HIV.

Pathology

1. ***Ulcerative:*** Multiple small ulcers coalesce to form large ulcers that may be thickened, infiltrated or everted with skip areas. They do not penetrate the muscularis mucosa, perforation is uncommon. The ulcers heal with extensive fibrosis leading to stricture, "Napkin ring appearance".
2. ***Hypertrophic type:*** Inflammation and fibrosis in submucosa mimicking a neoplasm.
3. ***Mixed variety:*** The mucosa has a cobblestone appearance with pseudopolyp, and flaps.
4. ***Diffuse:*** Resembling ulcerative colitis.

Granulomas in bowel and lymph node are usually caseating.

Clinical Features: Symptoms include nonspecific abdominal pain, weight loss, lassitude, distension of abdomen. ("Ball of Wind-gala"), constipation, diarrhea, occasionally bleeding. The pain in lower abdomen can be in the right, or left lower quadrant, crampy or colicky pain increases on eating and decreases by vomiting and defaecation. There is doughy feeling of the abdomen due to extensive fibrous adhesion and inflammation.

Treatment: Short course chemotherapy cures majority of the cases.

Complications: (1) Stricture formation with subsequent obstruction. (2) Luminal narrowing due to inflammation and adenitis, colonic traction, diverticula, fixation and sinus formation. (3) Fistula due to secondary bacterial infection. (4) Secondary malabsorption syndrome due to decreased absorptive area, bacterial overgrowth ("Stagnant loop syndrome").

Peritoneal TB: Constitute 4-10% of extrapulmonary TB. It may be due to activation of latent focus or hematogenous spread. Ascites occurs due to studding of parietal and visceral peritoneum by exudation or from contiguous nodes. There are three types: (1) **Ascitic type** or exudative type. (2) Plastic or **hyperplastic** type involving the greater omentum. (3) **Fibrotic** with focal and minimal fibroblastic with peritoneal adhesion.

Clinical Features: Common in females, insidious in onset. Symptoms include anorexia, abdominal distention, and doughy abdomen ("cotton wool sign"). Plastic form presents as a lump. Fibrotic form presents with features of obstruction.

Tabes Mesenterica

Glandular TB abdomen involving mesenteric nodes in children mimicking appendicitis. Children present with fever, intermittent abdominal pain, localised to right iliac fossa mimicking appendicitis.

Investigations: *USG Abdomen* which may show fixed membranes, septa, floating debris or omental cake; thickened mesentery with adherent loops, lymphadenopathy. CT scan of the abdomen may show high-density ascites with abdominal lymphadenopathy. Paracentesis shows straw colored exudative high proteineceous fluid with lymphocytic predominance which is classical of tuberculosis. Smear is positive for AFB in 3%. Culture positive in 10-20%. Increased ADA activity in ascitic fluid is sensitive and specific for TB peritonitis. But it may be diminished in HIV. Stool examination for AFB culture can be a useful addition. Barium study of the small intestine and colon may show: (1) Increased transit time with hyper segmentation and flocculation of barium (earliest sign). (2) Thickening of mucosal folds with scalloping speculation. (3) Ulceration. (4) Sterling sign: exclusion of barium from an involved segment with adjacent normal looking segments. (5) Fleishner's sign: ileocaecal valve is patulous in TB, stenotic in Crohn's. (Table 5.3 gives the histopathological differences between TB and Crohn's). Biopsy: either direct or laparoscopic/ USG or CT guided biopsy. Yield is nearly 60-75%.[4]

Table 5.3: Histopathological features

Histopathological features differentiating TB and Crohn's	TB	Crohn's
Granuloma surrounded by inflammation	+	—
Submucosal widening	—	+
Transmural/follicular hyperplasia	—	+
Epithelial regeneration	+	—
Glandular metaplasia	+	—

Treatment: Short course chemotherapy.

TB BRAIN

Tuberculosis of the brain occurs in 5-10% of adult cases of clinical TB and 20-60% of children dying with active TB have a brain or meningeal involvement. In India, TB meningitis constitutes nearly 50-55% of bacterial meningitis.

Bacteriology: Majority of cases is due to mycobacterium tuberculosis. NTM and bovine species contribute to less than 5%.[5]

TB Meningitis (TBM)

Pathology: TBM occurs in 3 stages: (1) Hematogenous seeding of the meninges "RICH FOCUS". (2) Quiescent phase for weeks, months. (3) Releasing phase which may be triggered by immune activation, coinfection, trauma which releases antigenic material into the meninges.

Progression and manifestation depends on: (1) Number of bacilli. (2) Virulence of the strain. (3) Immune status of the individual.

Meningeal Changes: Exudation occurs between pia and arachnoid thickening the arachnoid. This is mainly composed of fibrin and inflammatory cells with neutrophils in the early period followed by lymphocytes, plasma cells, epithelioid and giant cells subsequently.

Vascular Changes: All size of arteries are involved the terminal portion of ICA and the proximal portion of MCA in the sylvian fissure are commonly affected. Vertebro-basilar vessels usually escape.

Parenchymal Changes: Due to meningeal and vascular changes, there is vascular insufficiency, edema, hydrocephalus, portion of brain adjacent to meninges has "border zone reaction" of edema, perivasculitis and gliosis.

Hydrocephalus: It occurs if the patient survives for 4-6 weeks, reasons are: (1) Blockage of cistern with the exudates in acute phase. (2) Adhesive leptomeningitis. (3) Due to obstruction of CSF circulation. (4) Blockage of aqueduct.

Clinical Features: Clinical profile has changed due to: (1) Mass BCG vaccination. (2) Later onset of primary infection. (3) Malnutrition. (4) HIV/AIDS.

Stages: Prodromal phase *(in children)* of vague ill health, apathy, irritability, loss of appetite, nausea, abdominal pain, convulsions in less than 2 years and depression, behavioural changes, headache, fever, meningismus in adults.

Stages in TBM (modified by BMRC) Stage 1: Nonspecific symptoms, fully conscious and alert.

Stage 2: Meningismus, drowsiness, lassitude, cranial nerve palsy due to presence of thickened basilar exudates compounded by hydrocephalus. Most common is VI nerve palsy followed by III, IV and VII.

Stage 3: Advanced stage comprising stupor, systemic toxicity, gross paresis paralysis, seizures, choreoathetosis, and coma. Ophthalmic signs include choroidal tubercles, papilloedema and internuclear ophthalmoplegia.

Diagnosis: Chest X-ray may show active or healed lesion of pulmonary TB.

CT scan of brain may give valuable information regarding enhancing exudates.

Hydrocephalus, infarcts due to vascular obstruction, tuberculoma or miliary nodules Gadolinium enhanced MRI is more sensitive as peripheral lesions are better visualized.

Treatment: Short course chemotherapy (9-12 months).

Steroids are indicated in stage II and III. When there is significant cerebral edema, spinal cord disease and drug reaction.

Surgery is indicated: (1) In releasing hydrocephalus if ICT is life threatening. (2) Vision is compromised. (3) CT shows progressive increase in size of the ventricles in spite of treatment.

Prognosis depends on: (i) Age of onset. (ii) Stage of the disease. (iii) Malnutrition. (iv) Prior BCG vaccination. (v) Increased ICT. (vi) Encephalopathy. (vii) Inadequate, improper, irregular treatment. (viii) Drug resistance.[6]

Tuberculoma

A tuberculoma results when intracranial tubercles enlarge without rupturing into the subarachnoid space. Tuberculoma refers to aggregate of small granulomatous lesion in the parenchyma of the brain. Sometimes there is a paradoxical reaction or treatment with ATT resulting in enlargement due to inflammatory response originating from released antigen.[6]

Types:

1. *Tuberculoma en-plaque.*
2. *Cystic tuberculoma.*
3. *Tuberculous abscess.*

They usually present with signs and symptoms of raised intracranial tension, focal signs occur in 85% of supratentorial type with seizures, focal motor deficits. Unlike meningitis, fever and systemic symptoms are not common. CT of the brain may show a thick ring of enhancement surrounded by a punctuate central clearing representing the caseous centre of the lesion.

Treatment: Short course chemotherapy. Rarely surgery is required.

EXTRAPULMONARY TB IN HIV

The global prevalence of HIV is 40 million with 3 million deaths/year. In India, there are an estimated 5.1 million cases. TB enhances HIV replication by secretion of TNF alpha, destruction of CD4 cells and fastened release of virions from infected cells and increased apoptosis. HIV promotes TB by decreasing macrophage activating lymphocytes, decreasing CD4 cells and increasing tissue destruction. *Mycobacterium tuberculosis* by itself may contribute to immunosuppression shown by Ellner *et al.* 1989. TB remains the most common opportunistic infection among HIV positive patients in India. The clinical and radiographic features vary with the degree of immunosuppression."[9] There is a greater tendency for extrapulmonary forms as well as disseminated TB as immunity goes down.[10] Extrapulmonary involvement in AIDS patients may be high as 70%.[11]

The introduction of HAART has dramatically changed the survival rate in all opportunistic infections including TB. In patients with HIV and TB, Anti retroviral therapy (ART) can be instituted if CD4 is less than 50 cells and after the intensive phase if CD4 is between 50-200 cells. This is because the maximum side effects of ATT drugs usually occur during the first 2 months. However, ART has to be modified due to the interactions between rifampicin and nevirapine and rifampicin and other protease inhibitors.

Immunoreconstitution Syndrome (IRS)

The development of a paradoxical reaction of IRS should be considered in patients with: (1) Emergence or worsening of the clinical manifestations of tuberculosis with or without positive acid-fast bacilli smear or culture results obtained from the involved organs. (2) Exclusion of other potential causes of the symptoms and signs after an extensive diagnosis evaluation, particularly drug fever and other infections related or not with HIV; and (3) Exclusion of drug resistant tuberculosis or other causes that could explain the persistence or relapse of tuberculosis.

Often there is an aggravation of symptoms, flare up of the disease, radiological worsening on instituting ART. It usually occurs in the first 1-4 weeks after initiating ART. This kind of paradoxical reaction has been reported earlier in TB itself especially with tuberculomas of the brain and lymph nodes. As a rule, other infections and resistance should be ruled out first. After reasonably excluding other causes, steroids can be given and gradually tapered along with ATT preferably in a tertiary care unit. Termination of ATT or HAART is rarely required.

REFERENCES

1. Dwight A. Powell, TB lymphadenitis, Schlossberg, David, Monographs in Infectious Diseases, Tuberculosis, New York, Praeger, 1993:143-150.
2. Paul T Davidson and Enrique Fernandex, Bone and Joint Tuberculosis, Schlossberg, David, Monographs in Infectious Diseases, Tuberculosis, New York, Prager, 1993:165-176.
3. M. Natarajan, Bone and joint tuberculosis, M.N. Natarajan, Natarajan Textbook of Orthopaedics and traumatology, Madras, MN Orthopaedic Hospital, 1995;51-63.
4. Stuart Lewis, Steven Field, Intestinal and peritoneal TB, William Rom and Stuart Garay, Tuberculosis, Boston, Little Brown and Company 1996:585-597.
5. Neetha Mehta, Neutrotuberculosis, Prof. K.C. Mohanty, Indian Expertise in TB, Mumbai, Lupin 133-153.
6. Michaeal Henry, Roberts Holzman, TB of Brain Meninges and spinal cord, William Rom and Stuart Garay, Tuberculosis, New York, Lippincott Williams and Wilkins, 2004:445-464.
7. Rani Balasubramanian and Rajeswari Ramachandran, Management of Non-Pulmonary forms of tuberculosis: Review of TRC studies over two decades. *Ind J Pediatr* 2000;67:34-40.
8. Radin. Intraabdominal mycobacteria TB and MAC in patients with AIDS, distinction based on CT findings. *AJR* 1991;156:487-491.
9. Raviglone MC, Narain JP, Koc. A. HIV associated TB in developing countires Clinical feature, diagnosis and treatment. *WHO Bull OMS* 1992;70:515.
10. F Chaison RE, Schider GF, Theier CP, Rutherford GN, Echenberg F, Hopewell PC. TB in patients with Human Immunodeficiency Syndrome, Clinical features, response to therapy and survival. *Ann Rev Respir Dis* 1987;136:570-74.
11. Jandermen G, Mc Donald RJ, Manial T. Tuberculosis manifestation of AIDS. *JAMA* 1986;256:362-366.

Chapter six

Cutaneous Tuberculosis

Vikas Sharma

Cutaneous tuberculosis makes up a small proportion of all cases of extrapulmonary tuberculosis which, in its turn, constitutes only a small fraction, perhaps about 10%. Recently, attention has been focused on the resurgence of cutaneous tuberculosis in the temperate regions. Interestingly, tuberculosis has re-emerged in areas with a high prevelance of HIV infection. It is probable that impaired cell mediated immunity as a consequence of HIV infection results in the reactivation of persisters, the dormant strains of *Mycobacterium tuberculosis*.The advent of HIV has led to a 20% increase in incidence of extra-pulmonary tuberculosis in USA. Since cutaneous tuberculosis constitutes 1.5% of all cases of extra-pulmonary tuberculosis, it is natural that its incidence will increase proportionately and there is more likelihood that clinicians may encounter more of such cases in the near future.

ETIOLOGY AND PATHOGENESIS

Tuberculosis of the skin is caused by *M. tuberculosis, M. bovis,* and, under certain conditions, the *bacillus calmette-guérin (BCG)*, an attenuated strain of *M. bovis.* It is transmitted through inhalation, ingestion, or inoculation. Following infection,T-lymphocytes interact with mycobacterial antigens displayed on the surface of antigen presenting cells and release lymphokines, interleukins and interferons. These are then responsible for activation and expression of MHC class II antigens and interleukin-2 receptor on the T-lymphocytes. There is accumulation of macrophages and resultant granuloma formation at the site. Memory T cells generated during initial sensitization remain in circulation and in lymphoid organs for a long time.

The outcome of infection is dictated by a number of independent but interrelated factors, namely:

1. Sensitization status of the host to mycobacterial antigens.
2. Nature of immune reactivity (in terms of CMI) of host as a consequence of sensitization.

3. Route of infection.
4. Pathogenicity of the infecting mycobacterial strain.

EPIDEMIOLOGY AND INCIDENCE

Even though mycobacterial diseases are widespread and serious, the organisms are neither very virulent nor very infectious: only about 5 to 10 percent of infections with *M. tuberculosis* lead to disease; the rate is similarly low for *M. leprae* and is very much lower for the facultative pathogens. Tuberculosis of the skin also has a worldwide distribution; while more prevalent in regions with a cold and humid climate in the past, it now also occurs in the tropics. In European and North American countries, the incidence of skin tuberculosis has shown a steady decline over the past decades. This seems to be true for all countries and parallels the decreasing incidence of pulmonary tuberculosis. A sharp increase of mycobacterial infection has occurred with increasing migrations and with the advent of the AIDS epidemic.

Its two most frequent forms are lupus vulgaris and scrofuloderma; in the tropics, lupus vulgaris is rare, whereas scrofuloderma and verrucous lesions predominate. Lupus vulgaris is more than twice as common in women as in men, while tuberculosis verrucosa cutis is most often found in men. Generalized miliary tuberculosis is seen in infants (and adults with severe immunosuppression or AIDS), as is primary inoculation tuberculosis; scrofuloderma usually occurs in adolescents and the elderly, while lupus vulgaris may affect all age groups.

CLASSIFICATION OF CUTANEOUS TUBERCULOSIS

I. Inoculation tuberculosis (exogenous source)	Tuberculosis chancre Warty tuberculosis (verruca cutis) Lupus vulgaris (some)
II. Secondary tuberculosis (endogenous source)	
Contiguous spread	Scrofuloderma
Auto-inoculation	Orificial tuberculosis
III. Haematogenous tuberculosis	Acute miliary tuberculosis Lupus vulgaris (some) Tuberculous gumma
IV. Eruptive tuberculosis (the tuberculides)	
i. Micropapular	Licen scrofulosorum
ii. Papular	Papular or papulonecrotic tuberculides
iii. Papulo-nodular	Erythema induratum (Bazin)
iv. Nodular	Nodular vasculitis Erythema nodosum

Cutaneous tuberculosis may evolve either as primary (tuberculous chancre and acute miliary tuberculosis) or as secondary infection (lupus vulgaris, tuberculosis verrucosa cutis, scrofuloderma and tuberculosis cutis orificialis). Secondary tuberculosis manifests in a sensitized host. Infection by another strain of *Mycobacterium tuberculosis* results in "reinfection" tuberculosis, with lupus vulgaris or tuberculosis verrucosa cutis as its cardinal expression. Reactivation of the dormant "persister" mycobacteria, consequent to lowered CMI, is responsible for "reactivation" that usually is either scrofuloderma or tuberculosis cutis orificialis.

Secondary tuberculosis forms a continuous immunopathologic spectrum extending from lupus vulgaris through tuberculosis verrucosa cutis and scrofuloderma to tuberculosis cutis orificialis, although there is considerable overlap. Lupus vulgaris and tuberculosis verrucosa cutis represent the "high-immune" pole with active CMI and apparently normal humoral immunity, whereas scrofuloderma and tuberculosis cutis orificialis represent impaired CMI with predominantly humoral immune response.

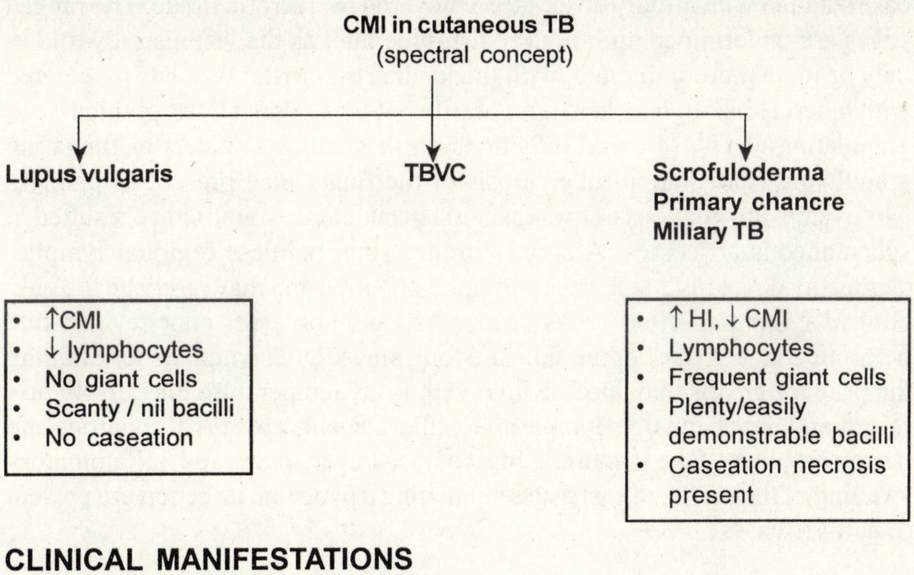

CLINICAL MANIFESTATIONS

Primary Inoculation Tuberculosis (Tuberculous Chancre; Tuberculous Primary Complex)

Tuberculous chancre is the result of the inoculation of M. tuberculosis into the skin of an individual without natural or artificially acquired immunity to this organism i.e. it results from the inoculation of mycobacteria into the skin of a host not previously infected with tuberculosis. The tuberculous chancre and the affected regional lymph nodes constitute the tuberculous primary complex of the skin.

Pathogenesis

Since tubercle bacilli cannot actively penetrate intact skin, they are introduced into the tissue at the site of minor abrasions or wounds. A rare "venereal" inoculation tuberculosis may occur in healthy individuals after sexual contact with patients suffering from genitourinary tuberculosis. Lesions in the mouth may be due to bovine bacilli from nonpasteurized milk and occur after mucosal trauma or tooth extraction. Primary inoculation tuberculosis following mouth-to-mouth resuscitation has been reported.The skin lesions appear 2 to 4 weeks after inoculation. Infection spreads to the regional lymph nodes, producing tuberculous lymphadenitis; with increasing acquired immunity, the process is localized to the particular region involved.

CLINICAL MANIFESTATIONS

The tuberculous chancre initially presents as a small papule, scab, or wound with little tendency to heal. A painless ulcer develops, which may enlarge to attain a diameter of over 5 cm. It is shallow with a granular or hemorrhagic base studded with miliary abscesses or covered by necrotic tissue. The ragged edges are undermined and of a reddish-blue hue; as the lesions grow older, they become more indurated, with thick adherent crusts. Wounds inoculated with tubercle bacilli may heal temporarily but break down later, giving rise to granulating ulcers. Mucosal infections result in painless ulcers or fungating granulomas. Inoculation tuberculosis of the finger may present as painless paronychia; inoculations of mycobacteria in puncture wounds have resulted in subcutaneous abscesses. A slowly progressing, painless regional lymphadenopathy develops 3 to 8 weeks after the infection and may rarely be the only clinical symptom. After weeks or months, cold abscesses may develop that perforate to the surface of the skin and form sinuses; the lymph nodes draining the primary glands may also be involved. Body temperature may be slightly raised and, occasionally, lymph node enlargement, abscess formation, and perforation may take a more acute course. Fever, pain, and inflammatory swelling of the surrounding tissues simulating a pyogenic infection are present in half the cases.

Histopathology

In the early phase, there is an acute inflammatory reaction and mycobacteria are easily detected. After 3 to 6 weeks, the infiltrate and the regional lymph nodes acquire a tuberculoid appearance.

Course

Without treatment, the condition may last upto 12 months. Lesions heal by scarring, but in rare cases lupus vulgaris develops at the site of a healed tuberculous chancre. In more than 50 percent of other cases the regional nodes calcify. Usually, the primary tuberculous complex yields satisfactory immunity, but reactivation of the disease may occur. Hematogenous spread may give rise to tuberculosis of other organs, particularly of the bones and joints. Depending on the size of the inoculum and the age and resistance of the host, primary inoculation tuberculosis may progress to acute miliary disease with fatal outcome.

TUBERCULOSIS VERRUCOSA CUTIS (WARTY TUBERCULOSIS)

An indolent, warty, plaque-like form of tuberculosis occurring as a result of the inoculation of organisms into the skin of a previously infected patient who usually has a moderate or high degree of immunity.

Pathogenesis

This is an inoculation tuberculosis occurring in persons who have acquired a certain degree of immunity. Thus, tests with PPD are highly positive. The inoculation of mycobacteria occurs at sites of minor wounds or abrasions. In the past, certain professional groups were most liable to acquire warty tuberculosis, particularly physicians, pathologists, medical students, and laboratory attendants, from tuberculous patients or from autopsy material ("verruca necrogenica", "anatomist's wart", "postmortem wart"). Farmers, butchers, and knackers contracted the disease from tuberculous cattle, and in these cases *M. bovis* was responsible. Children can become infected by playing and sitting on ground contaminated with tuberculous sputum.

CLINICAL FEATURES

Lesions occur on those areas exposed to trauma and infected sputum or other tuberculous material. The hand is most commonly involved in Europe, but the knees, ankles and buttocks in Eastern countries. The lesion starts as a small, symptomless, indurated, warty papule with a slight inflammatory areola. By gradual extension a verrucose plaque is formed. Irregular extension at the edges leads to a serpiginous outline with finger-like projections. The centre may involute leaving a white atrophic scar or the whole lesion forms a massive, infiltrated papillomatous excrescence (Fig. 6.1) . The colour is purplish, red or brown. The consistency is generally firm but there may be areas of relative softening.

Histopathology

The most prominent features are pseudoepitheliomatous hyperplasia with marked hyperkeratosis and dense inflammatory infiltrates. Abscesses form in the superficial dermis or within the pseudoepitheliomatous rete pegs. Epithelioid

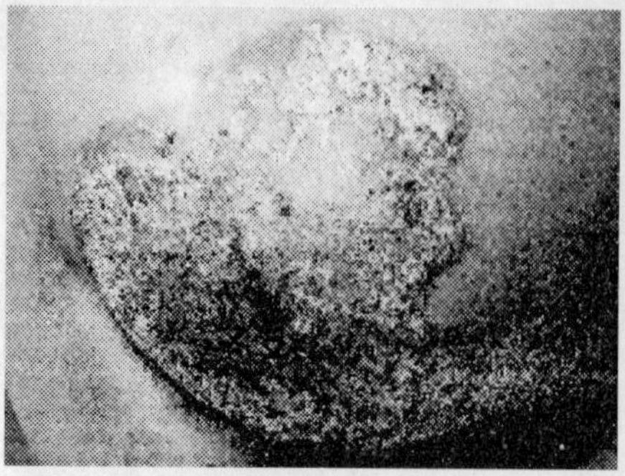

Fig. 6.1: Large plaque of tuberculosis verrucosa cutis ***(See also Colour Plate 2)***

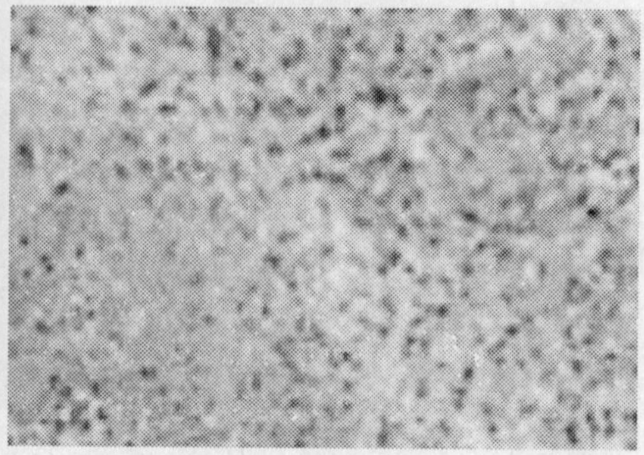

Fig. 6.2: Histopathology of TBVC showing well-ill defined tuberculoid granulomas surrounded by lymphocytes ***(See also Colour Plate 2)***

cells and giant cells are found in the midportions of the dermis and beneath the epidermis; typical tubercles may form but are uncommon (Fig. 6.2). Mycobacteria can be demonstrated occasionally. At times, the dermal infiltrate may be nonspecific.

Prognosis

The condition responds to antituberculosis treatment; without it, extension is usually extremely slow and lesions may remain virtually inactive for months or years. Spontaneous remission often occurs. Active disease of other organs should be looked for, as osseous, glandular or pulmonary tuberculosis may coexist.

Lupus Vulgaris

A progressive form of cutaneous tuberculosis occurring in a person with a moderate or high degree of immunity. The characteristic lesion is a plaque, composed of nodules of an 'apple-jelly' colour, which extends irregularly in some areas, while in others scarring occurs, causing considerable tissue destruction over many years.

Pathogenesis

Lupus vulgaris is a postprimary form of skin tuberculosis arising in previously sensitized individuals with only moderate immunity. The lesions progress steadily and, although spontaneous involution does occur, new lesions arise within old scars. Complete healing is only rarely observed without therapy. Lupus vulgaris originates from tuberculosis elsewhere in the body by hematogenous, lymphatic, or contiguous spread, most often from cervical adenitis or pulmonary tuberculosis, sometimes from an old, apparently quiescent primary complex. Rarely, it follows primary inoculation tuberculosis or BCG vaccination.

CLINICAL FEATURES

The lesions are usually solitary, but two or more sites may be involved simultaneously; in patients with active pulmonary tuberculosis, multiple foci may develop. In about 90 percent of patients the head and neck are involved. Lupus vulgaris usually starts on the nose or cheek and slowly extends onto adjacent areas. The earlobes are often affected, and solitary patches may be encountered on the scalp. Only a small percentage of the lesions occur on the extremities, and, except for cases with disseminated lupus vulgaris, involvement of the trunk is rare. In general, lupus vulgaris is asymptomatic. The initial lesion is the lupus macule or papule, characterized by a brownish-red color and a soft, friable consistency. Upon diascopy the infiltrate exhibits a typical apple-jelly color. Early lesions are small, rather ill-defined infiltrates with a smooth surface or covered by a scale. Progression is characterized by an elevation of the lesions and a deeper brownish color. Involution in one area and simultaneous expansion in another result in plaques with a gyrate outline. Its course is marked by ulceration and scarring; thus, its clinicalmanifestations are diverse and a number of complications may ensue.

Plaque Form

Extension occurs with little or no central scarring, and little infiltration. The distinctive colour may be masked by erythema (Fig. 6.3). Scaling may lead to a psoriasiform appearance, particularly on the legs. Large plaques with serpiginous or polycyclic margins may cover wide areas of the body. Irregular scarring leaves islands of activity which persist indefinitely. The edge often becomes thickened and hyperkeratotic.

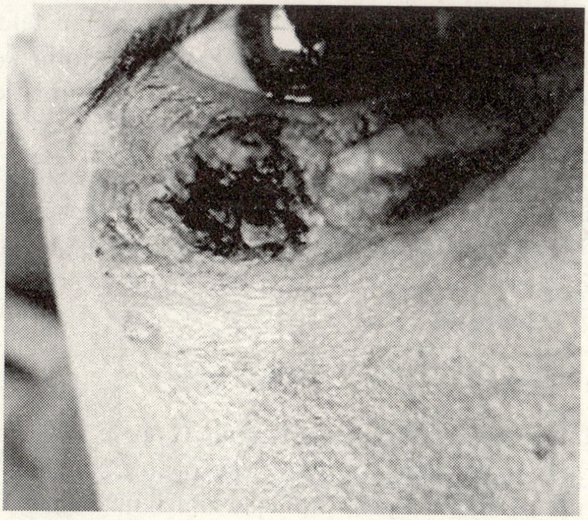

Fig. 6.3: Plaque lesion of lupus vulgaris showing central ulceration ***(See also Colour Plate 2)***

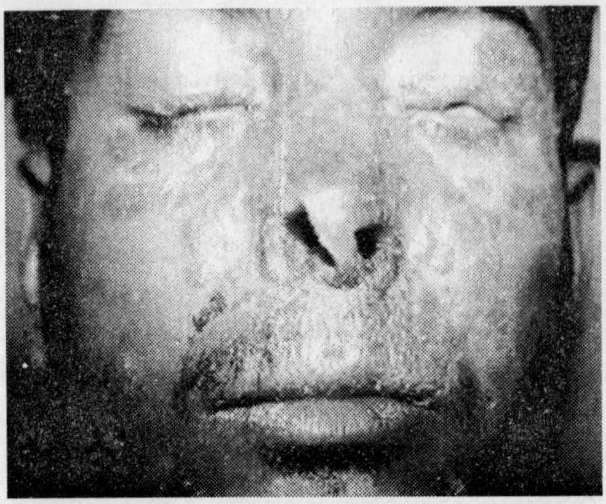

Fig. 6.4: Multiple, multicentric, papulo-nodulo-plaque lesions of lupus vulgaris distributed over– cheeks, malar area, nose, upper lip. Loss of both alae nasi, more so of left one can be noticed. Contractures of right upper eyelid with cicatricial ectropion are seen ***(See also Colour Plate 3)***

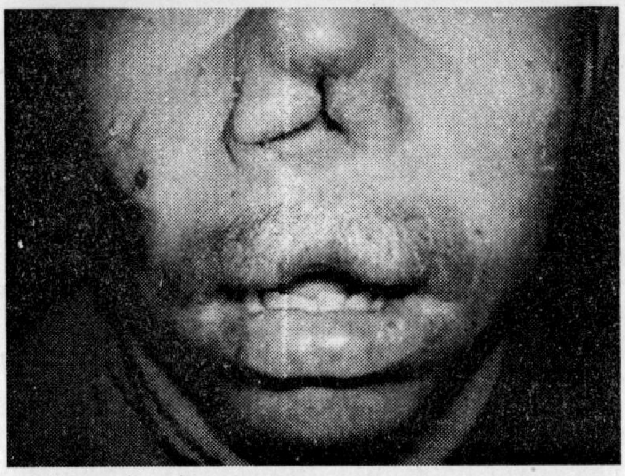

Fig. 6.5: Nodulo-plaque lesions of lupus vulgaris over nose and upper lip. Loss of both alae nasi can be seen, exposing posterior part of nasal septum. Upper lip is swollen and fissured ***(See also Colour Plate 3)***

Ulcerative and Mutilating Forms

Scarring and ulceration predominate. Crusts form over areas of necrosis. The deep tissues and cartilage are invaded, and contractures and deformities mask the progress of the disease (Figs 6.4 and 6.5). In the mild form, keratotic plugs overlying pin-point ulcers are associated with slow scar formation.

Vegetating Forms

A marked tendency to rate, often rapidly, produces areas of necrosis and phagedena. Infiltration is extensive but scarring is minimal. Mucous membranes are invaded and cartilage is slowly destroyed ('lupus vorax'). Response to chemotherapy is excellent.

Tumour-like Forms

These show the opposite characteristics and course. The lesion, deeply infiltrating, stands out from the skin as a group of soft, smooth nodules or as a more extensive, soft, reddish-yellow plaque which may be hypertrophic and evolves very slowly. Scaling and scarring are absent. In the 'myxomatous' form, huge soft tumours occur predominantly on the ear lobes which become grossly enlarged. Lymphoedema and vascular dilatation are sometimes marked. The response to treatment may be poor.

Papular and Nodular Forms

Multiple lesions occur in disseminate lupus-true 'miliary lupus'.

Lupus Vulgaris of Mucous Membranes

The nasal, buccal or conjunctival mucosa is involved in many cases and must be examined carefully. Nasal lesions start as nodules which bleed easily and then ulcerate, sometimes destroying the cartilage. After the apparent cure of skin lesions, nasal foci may proliferate and give rise to recurrences. Granulating, vegetating or ulcerating lesions of the buccal mucosa, palate, gingiva or oropharynx may occur by direct extension or by lymphatic spread from nasal lesions.

Lupus Postexanthematicus

Following a transient impairment of immunity, particularly after measles (thus the term lupus *postexanthematicus*), multiple disseminated lesions may arise simultaneously in different regions of the body due to hematogenous spread from a latent tuberculous focus. During and following the eruption, a previously positive tuberculin test may become negative but will usually revert to positive as the general condition of the patient improves. Clinically and histopathologically, the lesions of postexanthematic lupus are typical for lupus vulgaris, and this distinguishes the condition from acute miliary tuberculosis

Histopathology

The most prominent feature is the formation of typical tubercles. Secondary changes may be superimposed: epidermal thinning and atrophy or acanthosis with excessive hyperkeratosis or pseudoepitheliomatous hyperplasia. Non-specific inflammatory reactions may partially conceal the tuberculous structures (Fig. 6.6). Old lesions are composed chiefly of epithelioid cells and may be impossible to distinguish from sarcoidal infiltrates.

Course

Lupus vulgaris is extremely chronic, and without therapy its course usually extends over many years or even decades. Thus, adults or older patients have more extensive lesions than children. Although there are periods of relative inactivity, it is progressive and leads to considerable impairment of function and to disfiguration. Contractions result in a reduction of joint mobility, and ulceration and destruction of the cartilaginous structures of the face and scarring

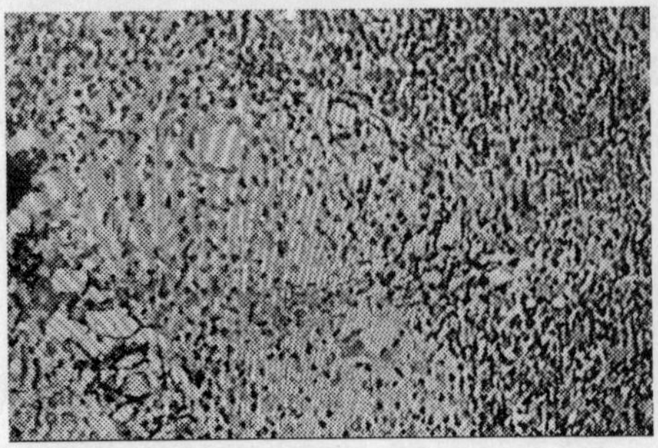

Fig. 6.6: Histopathology of lupus vulgaris. Epithelioid cell tubercles surrounded by dense lymphocytic infiltration but without caseation. There are some giant cells of the Langhans type ***(See also Colour Plate 3)***

lead to cicatricial ectropion with its complications, to microstomia with impairment of speech and food intake, and to other severe mutilations.The most serious complication of long-standing lupus vulgaris is the development of carcinoma. Early in this century this was estimated to occur in almost 10 percent of patients. Squamous cell carcinomas outnumber basal cell carcinomas by far, and the incidence of metastases is surprisingly high.

The Relationship of Lupus Vulgaris to Tuberculosis of Other Organs

In 40 percent of patients with lupus vulgaris there is associated tuberculous lymphadenitis, and 10 to 20 percent have pulmonary tuberculosis or tuberculosis of the bones and joints. The morbidity of lupus vulgaris patients from pulmonary tuberculosis is 4 to 10 times higher than in the general population. In some cases, lupus vulgaris may be regarded as a symptom of another tuberculous disease running a serious course.

SCROFULODERMA (TUBERCULOSIS COLLIQUATIVA CUTIS)

Scrofuloderma is a subcutaneous tuberculosis leading to cold abscess formation and a secondary breakdown of the overlying skin.

Pathogenesis

Scrofuloderma results from the involvement and breakdown of the skin overlying a tuberculosis focus, usually a lymph gland but sometimes an infected bone, joint or even a lacrimal gland or duct.

Histopathology

The histopathological changes are those of tuberculous granulation tissue. Caseation necrosis may be seen in the deeper dermis. Tubercle bacilli can usually be isolated from the pus.

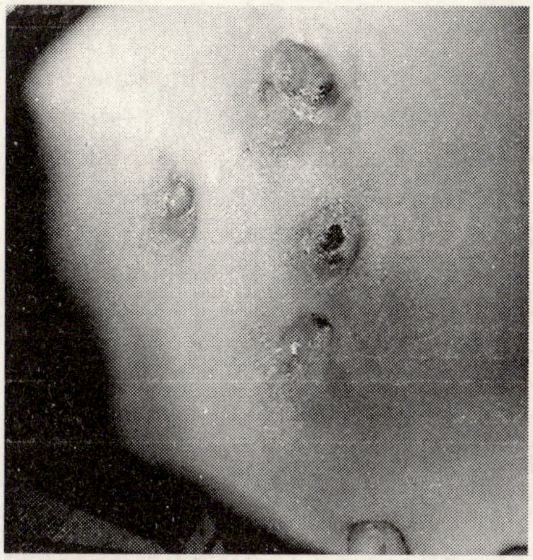

Fig. 6.7: Lesions of scrofuloderma *(See also Colour Plate 3)*

Clinical Features

A bluish red nodule overlying the infected gland or joint breaks down to form undermined ulcers with a floor of granulating tissue. Numerous fistulae may intercommunicate beneath ridges of a bluish skin. Progression and scarring produce irregular adherent masses, densely fibrous in places and fluctuant or discharging in others. Excessive granulation tissue may give rise to fungating tumours (Fig. 6.7). After healing, characteristic puckered scarring marks the site of the infection.

Course

Spontaneous healing does occur, but the course is very protracted and it may take years before the inflammatory and ulcerative lesions have been completely replaced by scar tissue. The typical scars permit a correct diagnosis, even after the process has become quiescent. Lupus vulgaris may develop at the site of scrofuloderma or in its vicinity.

METASTATIC TUBERCULOUS ABSCESS (TUBERCULOUS GUMMA)

Definition and Pathogenesis

The metastatic tuberculous abscess is due to hematogenous spread of mycobacteria from a primary focus during a period of lowered resistance, resulting in single or multiple cutaneous and subcutaneous lesions. It usually occurs in undernourished children of low socio-economic status or in immunodeficient or severely immunosuppressed patients; occasionally it may cause a carpal tunnel syndrome.

Clinical Manifestations

Subcutaneous abscesses, which are generally nontender and fluctuant, arise either singly or as multiples on the trunk, extremities, or head; the lesions may invade the overlying skin and break down, forming fistulas and ulcers. Metastatic tuberculous abscesses may occur with progressive organ tuberculosis or in miliary tuberculosis but may occur without any underlying tuberculous focus. Tuberculin sensitivity is usually lower than in other forms of skin tuberculosis and may be absent in severely ill patients.

Histopathology

As in scrofuloderma, massive necrosis and abscess formation are found. Acid-fast stains usually reveal copious amounts of mycobacteria.

Orificial Tuberculosis (Tuberculosis Ulcerosa Cutis et Mucosae)

Orificial tuberculosis is a rare form of tuberculosis of the mucous membranes and the skin of the orifices due to autoinoculation of mycobacteria from progressive tuberculosis of internal organs.

Pathogenesis

The underlying disease is far advanced pulmonary, intestinal, or, rarely, genitourinary tuberculosis. Mycobacteria shed from these foci in large numbers are inoculated into the mucous membranes of the orifices, usually after trauma. Most patients show a positive intradermal tuberculin reaction, but in terminal stages energy develops.

Clinical Manifestations

In orificial tuberculosis of the mouth, the tongue is most frequently affected, particularly the tip and the lateral margins, but the soft and hard palate are also common sites. In far-advanced cases the lips are also involved, and the oral condition often represents an extension of ulcerative tuberculosis of the pharynx and larynx. In cases with intestinal tuberculosis, lesions develop on and around the anus, and in females with active genitourinary disease, the vulva is involved. A small yellowish or reddish nodule appears on the mucosa and breaks down to form a circular or irregular ulcer with a typical punched-out appearance, undermined edges, and soft consistency. Its floor is covered by pseudomembranous material and often exhibits multiple yellowish tubercles and eroded vessels. The surrounding mucosa is swollen, edematous, and inflamed. Lesions may be single or multiple and are extremely painful. The tenderness is often out of proportion to the size of the ulcers and results in dysphagia and inability to eat.

Histopathology

There is a massive nonspecific inflammatory infiltrate and necrosis, but tubercles with caseation may be found deep in the dermis. Mycobacteria are easily demonstrated.

Course

Orificial tuberculosis is a symptom of advanced internal disease with a most unfavorable prognosis. Individuals developing orificial tuberculosis run a downhill course, and as the internal condition progresses, the orificial lesions enlarge and spread.

ACUTE MILIARY TUBERCULOSIS OF THE SKIN (TUBERCULOSIS CUTIS MILIARIS DISSEMINATA)

Definition and Pathogenesis

Miliary tuberculosis of the skin is an extremely rare skin manifestation of fulminating miliary tuberculosis due to hematogenous dissemination of mycobacteria. The initial focus of infection is either meningeal or pulmonary, and the disease may follow infections such as measles and HIV, which reduce the immunologic defense mechanisms; it most often occurs in babies and infants. Tuberculin sensitivity is usually absent.

Clinical Manifestations

Disseminated lesions occur on all parts of the body, particularly on the trunk. They consist of minute erythematous macules or papules and purpuric lesions. Sometimes unbilicated vesicles or a central necrosis and crust develop.

Histopathology

Initially, necrosis and nonspecific inflammatory infiltrates and small abscesses are prominent, and occasionally signs of vasculitis may be seen. Mycobacteria are present both in and around blood vessels. In later stages (if the patient develops immunity), lymphocytic cuffing of the vessels and even tubercles may be observed.

Course

The prognosis is poor, but a favorable outcome after treatment is possible.

The Tuberculides

The term tuberculide is applied to any of a group of eruptions which arise in response to an internal focus of tuberculosis and clear with antituberculosis therapy. They are usually symmetrical and disseminated.

Aetiology

Tuberculides are probably due to the haematogenous dissemination of tubercle bacilli in a person with a moderate or high degree of immunity; but the underlying focus of tuberculosis may not be clinically active at the time of the eruption, and the patient is often in excellent health. Fluctuations in the immunological state of the patient probably determine the development and features of the eruption, stasis, skin temperature and the relative blood supply being responsible.

LICHEN SCROFULOSORUM

Lichen scrofulosorum is a lichenoid eruption of minute papules occurring in children and adolescents with tuberculosis.

Clinical Manifestations

The eruption is asymptomatic and is usually confined to the trunk. The lesions consist of small, firm, follicular or parafollicular papules of a yellowish or pink color; they have a flat top or bear a minute horny spine or fine scales on their surface. Lichenoid grouping is pronounced and results in the formation of rough, discoid plaques that tend to coalesce. The lesions persist for months, but spontaneous involution eventually ensues. Antituberculous therapy results in complete resolution within a matter of weeks.

Histopathology

Superficial tuberculoid granulomas develop around hair follicles but may also occur independent of the adnexae. Mycobacteria are not seen in the sections and cannot be cultured from biopsy material.

Papulonecrotic Tuberculid

This is a symmetric eruption of necrotizing papules appearing in crops and healing with scar formation.

Clinical Manifestations

Sites of predilection are the extensor aspects of the extremities, buttocks, and lower trunk with a symmetric distribution. Disseminated crops of dusky red, symptomless, pea-sized papules appear. They may show a central depression and an adherent crust over a crater-like ulcer. If the lesions are seated more deeply, they may enlarge to a diameter of 1 cm and acquire a more livid color. There is spontaneous involution, and pitted scars result. Usually there are no systemic symptoms.

Histopathology

The most characteristic feature is a wedge-shaped necrosis of the upper dermis extending into the epidermis. The inflammatory infiltrate surrounding this necrotic area may be nonspecific but is usually tuberculoid. Involvement of the blood vessels is a cardinal feature and consists of an obliterative and sometimes granulomatous vasculitis leading to thrombosis and complete occlusion of the vascular channels. Recanalization of the vessels may be observed.

Erythema Induratum of Bazin

This is a chronic recurring nodular and ulcerative disorder of the lower legs.

It is usually localized to the legs of women but occasionally occurs in other areas and, rarely, in men.

DIAGNOSIS

The diagnosis of cutaneous tuberculosis is based on relative and absolute criteria, apart from other supportive immunological evidence.

Relative

i. *Characteristic history of evolution of the disease.*
ii. *Strongly positive Mantoux test.*
iii. *Characteristic histopathology.*
iv. *AFB in lesion.*
v. *Therapeutic response.*

Absolute

i. *Recovery of M. tuberculosis in culture on Lowenstein Jensen's medium after 4 to 6 weeks of inoculation.*
ii. *Recovery of M. tuberculosis on inoculation of material from lesions into guinea pigs.*
iii. *DNA identification by PCR (detects a 65KDa Ag) specific for M. tuberculosis.*
iv. *Rapid cultural assay–BACTEC system (2-6 days).*

MANAGEMENT

- Care of the patient as a whole.
- Rule out any other organ involvement with tuberculosis.
- Drug therapy :
  2 EHRZ + 4 HR (Recommended by British and American thoracic societies and WHO for new cases of severe extra-pulmonary TB)

2 HRZ + 6 HE (Recommended by WHO for new cases of less severe form of cutaneous TB)

HIV co-infection: 2 HREZ + 7HR or HR for 6 months following –ve culture reports.

Multidrug Resistant TB:

Incidence of Resistance to single drug (14%)

INH – 9% ; PYZ – 6%

RIF – 4% ; ETM – 2%

Treated by using 6-9 Antitubercular drugs.

Other Measures

- Surgical excision of small lesions of LV or TBVC.
- Local destruction (electro/cryo) of small residual nodules of LV.
- Surgical debridement in scrofuloderma which decreases the duration of ATT.
- Reconstructive surgery for disfigurement left by LV.

REFERENCES

1. Textbook of Dermatology—Fitzpatrick.
2. Textbook of Dermatology—Rook.
3. Dermatopathology—Lever.
4. International Journal of Dermatology—1990; 29.
5. International Journal of Dermatology—1994; 33: 02.
6. International Journal of Dermatology—1989;28: 04.
7. British Journal of Dermatology – 1988;118;730.

Chapter seven

TB of Serous Membranes

RS Bhatia

INTRODUCTION

Serosal involvement in tuberculosis is not uncommon. Fluid collection is quite commonly seen in routine practice, the number of cases involved is increasing because of increasing number of HIV co-existing with TB. Drug management with present day anti-TB chemotherapy is sufficient to treat these cases. Surgery is rarely indicated when complicated.

TUBERCULOUS PLEURAL EFFUSION

Pleural affection and effusion in tuberculosis are the most common affliction in high TB prevalence regions. Incidence is increased with coexisting HIV disease. Pleural involvement may occur as a part of primary TB in children, and young adults with pyrexia and pleurisy or as a part of disseminated TB in AIDS patients. Pathogenesis of pleural effusion involves delayed type of hypersensitivity, that occurs due to release of tuberculous protein into the pleural space following the rupture of subpleural caseous focus into the pleural space. Local inflammatory reaction occurs because of release of cytokines such as IL2, IL1, TNF alfa, IL6, IL10, IL12 and IFNy by the activated lymphocytes and macrophages. Lymphocytes in the pleural fluid are in a ratio of CD4: CD8:: 3:4. Pleural fluid culture for mycobacterium tuberculosis is most of the time non-contributory (negative). PPD skin test may be negative in one third of the cases, possibly due to circulating adherent cell which suppresses the specifically sensitized circulatory T lymphocytes in the peripheral blood or due to sequestration of PPD reaction T lymphocytes in the pleural space.

Clinical manifestations include fever, chest pain and non-productive cough in almost three fourth of the cases, and these patients, generally 1/3rd; reach the family physician within a week's time. Those with chronic infection, generally 2/3rd of cases, present with malaise, dyspnoea and weight loss, within a month's period. Rarely, patient may present in a critically sick situation with polyserositis, afflicting multiple serosal involvement. Tuberculosis pleural effusion is generally unilateral and is of moderate degree. In primary TB, effusion may be present without any evidence of lung parenchymal disease, while lung parenchyma may be accompanying the effusion in post-primary (reactivation) tuberculosis. Negative tuberculosis test initially in one third of cases generally becomes positive after 6-8 weeks. Therefore, negative test does not rule out tuberculous pleuritis. Plain X-ray chest may show tubercular parenchymal infiltration accompanying pleural effusion in one third of cases. Aspirated fluid is never bloody, mostly serosanguinous, testing proteins > 5 gm/dl and glucose < 60 mg/dl. Cellular analysis may show polymorphs in early phase (with 7-10 days) but later on predominantly small lymphocytes are seen. Eosinophils rarely exceed 10%, mesothelial cells are rare and if more the 5%; this disfavors the diagnosis of TB. ADA levels of >70 IU/L has 98% and 96% of sensitivity and specificity respectively. However, ADA levels may go down to < 40 IU/L in immuno compromised patients. Pleural fluid interferon level > 200 pg/ml, favours the diagnosis of TB. Sensitivity and specificity of 81% and 78% respectively of PCR is diagnostic TB aetiology. Demonstration of mycobacterium tuberculosis in the fluid from pleural cavity is possible in < than 10% of cases. Three different pleural biopsy specimens may increase the diagnosis yield from 60-100%. Presence of granuloma in parietal pleura, without the demonstration of caseous necrosis and AFB, is suggestive of diagnosis although granuloma may be present in other diseases such as fungal, RA, and tularemia. Short course anti-tuberculosis treatment is sufficient to treat these patients. Corticosteroids are only indicated for acute symptoms and should be rapidly tapered off as soon as patient responds.

Therapeutic thoracocentesis has not been indicated, and decortication is only considered, when there is empyema; extra pleural pneumonectomy and thoracoplasty are also recommended.

TUBERCULAR PERITONITIS

Peritoneal involvement in tuberculosis can occur secondary to abdominal tuberculosis, but it is more commonly affected by haematogenous spread from foci in the lungs. Most common variety is exudative peritonitis leading to ascites, other varieties include encysted or loculated type, fibrous or plastic type and rarely purulent type of TB peritonitis. Higher incidence of 3% of tubercular peritonitis has been reported in patients of end stage renal failure on dialysis. Diagnosis is made on the basis of positive AFB culture of dialysate.

The onset is insidious in almost three fourth of cases, taking 3-4 months, presenting with fever, anorexia, weight loss and abdominal pain and a mass in fibroadhesive variety. Abdominal examination gives a tender and doughy feel. Shifting dullness in ascites is present except when the fluid is loculated. Ascitic fluid tap may demonstrate total proteins > 3.0 g/dl. SAAG is < 1.1. Lymphocytes, AFB are rarely demonstrable, fluid culture is positive for AFB in 20% of cases. ADA is highly specific for tuberculous ascites. Mantoux test is usually positive. CT abdomen may reveal local pathology of thickened blood, lymphadenopathy, genital affection in females and CT guided biopsy of the lesion may reveal caseating granuloma in > 90% of cases. Chest X-ray may be positive for tuberculous pathology in case of haematogenous spread from foci in the lungs. Short course anti-tuberculous treatment is effective. Those who continue to experience symptoms of bowel obstruction, may need surgery to release the adhesions.

TUBERCULOUS PERICARDITIS

A rising trend from 0.4% to highest trend of 11% in acute pericarditis has been observed in tuberculous pericarditis in the last five decades all over the world, the effect may be due to resurgence of tuberculosis due to AIDS in the past two decades. Indian tuberculous pericarditis has been reported to have prevalence rate of 3.3% in cases of chronic pericardial effusions. Tuberculous pericarditis occurs in 1-2% of cases of pulmonary tuberculosis. Disease mostly spreads from local tracheobronchial, mediastinal or hilar nodal lesions; haematogenous spread from lungs and other organs can also occur. Initial deposit of pericardial fibrin is associated with serosanguinous or even blood stained effusion, that occurs because of hypersensitive reaction to tubercular protein. In subacute stage, granulomatous pericardial inflammation is followed by infiltration of epithelioid histocytes and Langhan's giant cells with caseating necrosis. In chronic (adhesive) phase, there is pericardial (both visceral and parietal) thickening with fibroblastic proliferation, that assumes a pattern of effusion constrictive pericarditis, if there is persistent effusion. In the later stage, obliteration of pericardial cavity without effusion may occur, eventually with pericardial calcification in developing frank constrictive pericarditis. Involvement of myocardium by mycobacterium (as mycocarditis) and developing cardiac temponade are future associated complications. However, lower incidence of cardiac temponade is expected in cases of dual infection of TB and AIDS, since AIDS may blunt the inflammatory response to tubercle bacilli.

Clinical presentation with a typical slow onset and accidental finding of large pericardial effusion is not uncommon, mostly seen in 3rd to 5th decades of life. Children and immunocompromised persons may present with acute pericarditis, cough, dyspnoea, fever, weight loss, chest pain, and ankle oedema (especially in cardiac temponade or constrictive pericarditis resulting in raised systemic venous pressure) and pain right upper quadrant due to hepatic congestion. Clinically silent disease with ascitis and hepatic congestion may mimick cirrhosis (Pick's disease). Eight different syndromes have been described; such as acute painful pericarditis, silent large effusion, cardiac temponade, acute pericardial constriction, subacute constriction, chronic constriction, pericardial calcification and undiagnosed pyrexia with eight loss and malaise. Pericardial pain and rub is seen in few patients. Exertional dyspnoea may be present in a patient with large effusion or associated pleural effusion (polyserosal affection). Symptoms of cardiac temponade or constrictive pericarditis are similar to those caused by other diseases. Patient is febrile, has tachycardia, hepatomegaly and cardiomegaly, with pulsus paradoxus. An ispiratory swelling of the neck veins (Kussmaul's sign) may be seen in patients with constrictive pericarditis. A pericardial knock can also be heard. Raised JVP, pulsus paradoxus and hypotension are present in patient with cardiac temponade which is attended as medical emergency.

Chest X-ray reveals pulmonary infiltrates in one third to three fourth of patients. Pericardial or effusive constrictive pericarditis is seen in almost 95% of cases as enlarged cardiac silhouette. Accompanying pleural effusion may be present in three fourth of cases. Pericardial calcification, though very rare, always pointer towards tubercular aetiology. ECG shows low voltage tracings. Electrical alternans may suggest cardiac temponade. Atrial fibrillation may occasionally be present. Pericardial fluid is serosanguinous or thickly bloody and has high protein content, and increased leukocytes contents, mainly lymphocytes. However, polymorphs may predominate in early phase (first 1-2 weeks). AFB smear positivity is upto 40%, culture positivity is upto 60% and guinea pig inoculation may yield 80% AFB positivity. Echocardiogram is non-contributory, CT scan and MRI give information about effusion and thickening of pericardium. PPD skin test is positive in 75-100% of cases; a negative PPD skin test is observed in 60% of cases with AIDS. False positivity of test is seen in one third of cases of idiopathic pericarditis whereas false negative test is observed in one fourth of cases of tuberculosis pericarditis. Value of adenosine deaminase activity of > 45 U/L has been 100% sensitive and 97% specific for tuberculous pleural fluid, has not been found applicable to tuberculous pericardial fluid.

Anti Koch's treatment with 3-4 drugs regimen is sufficient to treat tuberculous pericarditis; corticosteroids when added, reduce the mortality and the need for pericardiocentesis but do not lessen the need for operation for constrictive pericarditis. Pericardiectomy is recommended only in selected cases of tuberculous pericarditis.

REFERENCES

1. Amrapurkar D; Abdominal TB in India; IN; S Das; ed. Med. Update API 2003;13:108-11.
2. Parel KA, Patel Ka; HIV and TB; IN, SB Gupta; ed. Med. Update; API 2005;15:726-730.
3. Richard W Light ; Pleural effusion; NEJM 2002;346;1971-77.
4. Balal R, *et al.* Site specific incidence of abdominal TB, Ind J. Gastroenterol 2000;19 (Supp-2): A44.
5. Rau NR, Serosal TB, IN, S Das; ed. Med. Update, API 2003;13:112-19.

6. Bhatia RS, TB and AIDS; JAPI 2000;48:613-16.
7. Bhatia RS, Diagnostic value of ELISA and ADA in TB; JAPI 1998;46:574.
8. Bhatia RS and Nigam P; Pulmonary TB—An Update; Curr. Med. Journ; 1997;3(5):19-24.
9. Bhatia RS; Update management of pulmonary tuberculosis; The Ind. Pract 1991;527-32.
10. Keane WF; *et al.* Adult peritoneal dialysis related peritonitis treatment recommendations; 2000 update; Perit Dial Int; 2000;20:396-411.
11. Pitchenik AE, Rubinson HA; The radiographic appearance of TB in patients with AIDS and pre-AIDS; Am Rev Resp Dis; 1985;131:393-96.

Chapter eight

Genitourinary Tuberculosis

BS Aulakh, RS Bhatia

INTRODUCTION

Genitourinary tuberculosis is ten times higher in patients with chronic renal failure. At the same time, bilateral renal tuberculosis can lead to renal failure.[1] Renal TB is due to haematogenous spread from primary infection, usually taking 5 to 10 years to develop, after the first infection. Renal tuberculosis accounts for 15-33% of all extrapulmonary TB. Incidence in HIV infected cases is almost 20% and in non-HN patients it is more than 9%.[2] Usually in affects only one side, and is not commonly seen in children. Disease affects kidney cortex, destroys the renal tissue as it spreads, forming a cavity. Further destruction may occur due to back pressure caused by obstruction by inflammatory material. Disease may spread to ureter, bladder and genitalia.

CLINICAL PRESENTATION

Cystitis, haematuria and lumbar pain are frequent symptoms.[3,4] Patient has increased frequency of passing urine, may be painful, with pain in the loin region and may present with painless haematuria. Renal tumour and bilharziasis are differential diagnosis. Sometimes patient may pass pus in urine and if culture is negative for non-tuberculosis bacteria, TB should be the likely diagnosis. Loin abscess is seen in late stage of the disease. Exceptionally, acute and chronic renal failure may occur.

DIAGNOSIS

Routine urine examination may not be of much help. Culture for mycobacterium, though may take some weeks, is reliable method. Plain KUB may show calcified, enlarged and distorted 'cummulous cloud' or 'cement kidney'. Intravenous pyelogram contributes towards diagnosis. IVP may show irregular shaggy calyces giving 'Moth eaten appearance or hydrocalyx or obliterated calyces or hydronephrosis, or non-functional kidney or hydroureter or small constricted bladder called 'Thimble bladder'. Cystoscopy may reveal 'Golf hole orifice'. Chest X-ray may rarely pointer towards primary infection. Renal dysfunctions can be judged from blood urea. PCR for tuberculosis helps in early diagnosis of genitourinary tuberculosis.

TB of Female Genitalia

Being an important cause of infertility in Asian countries, almost 10% infertile females and 1% of patients attending gynaecology OPD in India are suffering from tuberculosis. Spread is by haematogenous route; lymphatic and contiguous organs spread has also been reported. In 50 to 80% of patients uterus is affected; fallopian tubes are also involved.

Clinically, infertility is the most common cause. Almost 10% of patients who suffered from TB in adolescence, have genitalial involvement. Almost 1/5th of cases give history of contact. A virgin with pelvic infection should be suspected of suffering from tuberculous genitalial infection. History of lower abdominal pain, malaise, fever and disturbed menstrual cycle in almost one third of cases is present. Nearly one fourth of cases show large abdominal masses due to fallopian tube abscess. However, pelvic examination may be normal in half the number of cases.

TB OF MALE GENITALIA

Individual or joint infection of prostrate, seminal vesicles and epididymis may occur, mostly from blood stream and from urinary tract.

Patient complains enlargement in scrotal sac, due to epididymis involvement, which is hard and craggy. Abscess may be formed and may find a route to skin as sinus. Prostrate and seminal vesicles may give craggy feel in nearly half the number of cases. Less than half percentage of patients may present with accompanying urinary symptoms.

Epididymal tumour can well be differentiated by hard feel, fever, chilly and acute pain locally differentiates acute epididymitis.

Treatment remains essentially the same, with initial four drug regimen for two months, followed by two drugs rifampicin and isoniazid for nine months. Drugs' dosage has to be adjusted according to creatinine clearance in case of renal failure, especially for streptomycin, ethambutol and isoniazid. In case of acute renal failure, ethambutol has to be dispensed 8 hours before haemodialysis. Ofloxacin added to the regimen offers good results.

Rifampicin has to be avoided in post renal transplant patients, as it increases the clearance of cyclosporin. Complicated renal abscess often has higher mortality in immuno suppressed patients.[5] Corticosteroids may help in preserving renal functions in tubercular interstitial nephritis.[6]

REFERENCES

1. Gusmao L *et al.:* Tuberculosis and kidney; Acta Med Port; 1998;11:1107-11.
2. Gopal R *et al.:* Extrapulmonary TB—A retrospective study; Ind J TB: 2001;48:225-26.
3. Gokcalp A *et al.:* Genitourinary TB—A review of 83 cases; Brit J Clin Pract; 1990;44:599-600.
4. Narayana AS: Overview of renal TB: Urology; 1982;19:231-37.
5. Jaik NP *et al.*: Renal abscess; JAPI; 2006;54:241-43.
6. Al-Suliman MH: *et al.*: Tuberculosis interstitial nephritis after—renal transplant; Transplantation; 1990;50:162-63.

Chapter nine

Tuberculosis and Lung Cancer

JS Sekhon and Amit Dhiman

Tuberculosis is a very common disease in developing countries and has been draining health care resources of these countries for a long time. Not only clinical but subclinical infections are also very common which may become dormant on their own. Tuberculosis lesions when they heal leave behind a lot of scar tissue and it was believed that squamous cell carcinoma may develop in these lesions.

However no study was done in an organized or planned manner to confirm this hypothesis. One of the problems was that patients would have to be followed up prospectively for years on end to detect if they develop carcinoma in a previously treated area of lung. Retrospective analysis as such do not answer this question.

Tuberculosis and lung cancer are known to coexist in endemic areas and have been reported frequently from Japan, Taiwan, China and India. In a study published from Japan by Tamara A *et al.* in May 2005, 61 cases of coexisting tuberculosis and lung cancer were detected at Tokyo National Hospital from 1991 to 2003. Majority was caused by Mycobacterium tuberculosis but other mycobacteria like mycobacterium kansani were also seen in a large proportion of patients. In a study from Madras 11 cases of coexisting tuberculosis and lung cancer were reported over 10 years period from 1980 to 1991. However the diagnostic criteria were not always culture positivity but a granuloma formation or appearance of cavitating lesions was also taken as confirmation.

Recently some date from China has emerged about the loss of heterozygosity (LDH) of Fragile Histidine Triad (FHIT). The authors used PCR based micro satellite analysis from micro dissected tissue and looked for FHIT protein expression that had long standing tuberculosis and had developed lung cancer in 40 patients from 1999 to 2003. The loss of heterozygosity of FHIT was found in 40% of patients with more than two years history of tuberculosis and none of patients with less than one year history of tuberculosis had loss of heterozygosity of FHIT zone. In patients with more than two years history of tuberculosis and lung cancer the cancer lesions showed loss of heterozygosity in more than 85% of lesions. Which was statistically significantly high as compared to lung cancer lesions with no past history of tuberculosis.

This is a path breaking study and employing the latest molecular techniques trying to establish a link between tuberculosis and lung cancer. This has circumvented the need to do prospective studies. However this study needs to be done on a larger scale and results need to be replicated. This does not circumvent the need to develop more molecular targets which can better establish a link and answer a question. Which has been bothering the developing world whether a link exists or not. For the time being it is an open question.

Chapter ten

Non-Radiological Diagnosis of the Tuberculosis

Jai Kishan, Navjot Pal Singh Bhullar

The diagnosing tuberculosis could be made without imaging the patient. CXR is not specific for tuberculosis. Even in RNTCP more emphasis is given on sputum examination than CXR.

The non-radiological diagnosis could be made with the help of:

1. History including nationality of patient (prevalence) of the disease in country where patient is living.
2. (i) Area of living, (ii) Detail feature of symptoms:
   - Sputum examination
   - MX test
   - Serology
   - Bectec
   - PCR
   - ADA
   - Etc.

Clinical History

1. **Family history:** Family history mainly concerned with history of contact at home. Heredity influence is not totally denied family history important when the index case is sp. +ve. Particularly to infants and children a history of contact with a sp. +ve case is a strong evidence in tuberculosis nature of illness.
2. **Past history:** Included any prolonged illness which may have decreased immunity and any treatment e.g. Steroids etc. makes patient more vulnerable to get infection with tuberculosis whoopy cough. Influenza appears to have strong potentiality to reactivate tuberculosis due to lowering of resistance.
3. **Occupational history:** Some occupation is injurious like when workers are exposed to dust. Silicon dust is known to have injurious effect where chance of tuberculosis may be more.

4. **Personal history:** Defective nutrition, excessive drinking a smoking, indifferent family life, late nights, inadequate rest, in short leading a desultory and irresponsible life—undermines health and resistance.
5. **History of present illness:** History of present illness is very important. Patient should be allowed to tell his/her complaints in his/her own words. You can assess his intelligence, his attitude towards illness etc.

The symptoms of pulmonary tuberculosis remain most rewarding basis of diagnosis.

Symptoms include:

1. General or constitutional symptoms.
2. Local symptoms.
3. Extrapulmonary symptoms.

General or Constitutional Symptoms

These are due to liberation of products from diseased foci into the blood stream and include lassitude, loss of weight, psychological symptoms, digestive disturbance, fever, tachycardia, amenorrhoea etc.

- Lassitude is one of the earliest symptoms in the beginning expressed only towards end of the day and gradually increases.
- Loss of appetite is slow but progressive is frequently seen.
- Symptoms of psychogenesis are occasionally seen in early phase.
- As a sure every case of active pulmonary tuberculosis exhibit some degree of pyrexia. In the early phases the fever is slight and occurs in the rate afternoon. On some day there may not be fever. So it should be recorded for few days. Some time fever may be high grade. Pulse rate is raised in proportion to lamp. Amenorrhoea in young unmarried girl is occasionally a presenting feature.

Local Symptoms

These are due to local disease caused by action of tuberculosis and include cough, haemoptysis, chest pain and dyspnoea.

Cough is most common and always the first to appear. Any copy more than 3 weeks of duration could be due to tuberculosis. Dry hacking cough may be seen in early phase. Followed by usually scanty or mucopurulent sputum.

Haemoptysis is very important diagnostic evidence. Although there are other causes also but tuberculosis is by far the most common cause.

Pain Chest: Although not a permanent feature but could be seen in case of dry pleurisy.

Extrapulmonary Symptoms

These are due to concurrent tuberculosis foci else where in the body important organs or sites involved are pleura, lymph gland, CNS, bones, skin etc., cold abscess, GIT etc.

Physical Signs: Through examination of patient may reveal general condition of patient and some signs of tuberculosis like scar mark, fistula or abscess etc. apart for cyanosis, clubbing, anaemia or pedal oedema may be seen.

Coolidge tube cannot supplant Lannec's tube. X-ray cannot diagnose chronic bronchitis pleural rub, pericardial friction, bronchial spasm, localized wheeze or rhonchus etc.

Physical examination should be done in detail and in systemic manner from inspection, palpation and percussion to auscultation.

Inspection may show kyphosis, poor expansion, scoliosis, and asymmetry of chest wall. Retraction, prominence etc. Diminished movements indicate the side involved or diseased.

Palpation: Displacement of trachea and apex beat may indicate some pathology palpation of lymph gland may also give due hint. Tactile vocal framitis are also helpful.

Percussion: Percussion node is dull over consolidation, strong dull on effusion and hyper resonant on pneumothorax. Shifting dullness may indicate hydropneumothorax.

Auscultation: Apart from normal vesicular breathing, tubular, amphoric or cavernous may be heard. Added sounds like crept or honcho all give some clue towards final diagnosis. Vocal resonance, whispering pectoriloquy or ego phony indicates consolidation.

Post tussive suction is heard due to the cavity. Post tussive rales are early sign of tuberculosis.

Lab. Diagnosis

Types of specimen used are:

1. Sputum—Pathological material expectoration.
2. Laryngeal swab—Charged with bronchial secretion.
3. Gastric lavage—Aspirated in the morning from fasting stomach.
4. Urine—Either 24 hours or early morning sample.

Lab. Techniques

Microscopic examination: Two methods usually used for staining are:

1. Ziehl—Nelson method.
2. Fluorescent method (Aura mine-Phenol method)

Fundamentally principle is same in both methods i.e. to demonstrate that bacilli are seen under microscope. False positive and false negative results are negligible, straining process is simpler and whole procedure completed in 5 minutes.

Concentration of specimen for microscopy: Smear examination can also be done after concentration of specimen where number of bacilli is supposed to be less. Sputum, thick pus, gastric juice is treated with 4% sodium hydroxide 2 : 1 ratio, incubated an hour and then centrifuged. CSF and serous fluid are prevented from clotting by adding a sterile citrate and then concentrated by centrifugation.

Sputum induction: Sputum smear examination result may be improved by sputum induction method where not enough sample of sputum is produced. The person is nebulized with warm saline or with medicines e.g. salbutamol, ambroxil etc.

Culture method: Although there are many methods of culture of tuberculosis but two methods, which are popularly used, are:

1. Dorset egg medium.
2. Lowenstein—Jensen method.

Usually inoculation on 2LJ slopes and 2 Dorset's egg medium slopes are done. The media slopes are heavily seeded caps are screed on tight to prevent evaporation of water and moisture essential for growth of tuberculosis. Petroff's method (Modified) is a concentration method to inoculated bacilli for culture.

Sward culture (nagon) method is used for sputum swab or laryngeal swap. Swabs are proved with 5! Oxalic acid unto 2/3rd of tube. Then fluid is transferred to 5% sterile sodium citrate of then swab is rubbed on medium (LD).

Animal inoculation: Guinea pigs are highly susceptible to both human and bovine bacilli. Certain materials like CSF, catheterized urine, pleural fluid can be centrifuged and directly inoculated without decontamination other materials are treated first as done for culture and then inoculated.

The following results may be noted in positive animals:

1. A local caseous lesion.
2. Enlargement of femoral, inguinal submandibular, portal, mediastinal and cervical lymph nodes with caseation.
3. Enlargement of spleen with presence of irregular necrotic areas.
4. Yellowish green necrotic areas in liver.
5. A few discrete tuberculosis in lungs.
6. **Other lab tests used are:**
   - Niacin test.
   - Catalase and peroxidase test.

Mantoux Skin Test (Tuberculosis Test)

This is a hypersensitivity test. Nearly all persons with either latent or active tuberculosis infection reacts positively to tuberculin. It is more useful in children.

Serological diagnosis of tuberculosis: In this test the circulating antibodies toward tuberculosis bacilli are tested. Some of these tests are:

A. *Agglutination of particles coated with antigen:*

1. **Middlebrook and dubos (1948) passive haemagglutination test**—In this human or sheep RBC's are coated with TB proteins and are agglutinated with patients serum.

2. Takahashi list (1962) here kaolin particles coated with methanol extract or tubercle bacilli were agglutinated with antisera of patient.
3. Latex particle can also be used instead of kaolin.
4. PPD linked to RBC by bio-diagozted bengindine was agglutinated with Igle or 75 antibodies of TB patient with active and inactive disease and of healthy controls.

B. *Double diffusion on agar gel:* Here gel diffusion method is applied 84% positively is recorded.

C. *Radio immune assays:*

i. **Determination of binding capacity** of IBI labelled extracts of TB bacilli has been described. IgG and Igm antibodies titers were determined and the binding ratio of both expressed. The extent of disease.

ii. **Immune fluorescent antibody technique:** In this serum from the patient is mixed with goat antihuman IgG antibody conjugated with fluorescent isothiocyanate and culture of TB bacilli on a slide. 96% of patient of TB show (+) and 7.5 of non-TB patient show (–) results.

1. **Radiometric methods:**

- **Bactec:** This system used fatty acid substrates like palmitic acid or formic acid labelled with radioactive CO_2. As mycobacteria utilize fatty acids, Radioactive CO_2 released which is measured as marker.
- **Mycobacteria growth indicator tubes (MGIT):** Smarter rapid method MGIT contains sound bottom tubes containing 4 ml of modified middle brook 7H9 broth which has an O_2 sensitive fluorescent sensor on the bottom. When mycobacterium grows the O_2 is reduced sow indicated to fluorescence brightly in 365 nm ultraviolet light.
- **Luciferase reporter assay** is another method, which is used for drug resistance tuberculosis.
- **Biochemical markers adenosine deamine activity (ADA)** is an amino hydrolase that catalyse the deamination of adenosine to inosine. Elevated levels of ADA are seen in tuberculosis effusions.

Polychain Reaction (PCR)

This is molecular biological method. With this technique a sequence of DNA can be amplified by using thermos aquaticus polymerase to the extent that it may be analyzed directly even from a minute amount of starting material PCR is extremely sensitive and specific technique.

Bromide partition test: Radioactive bromide partition test is used for the early diagnosis of TB meningitis. The partition of bromide between serum and CSF after a loading close reflects the integrity of the blood brain barrier.

Gas chromatography: Gas chromatography of mycobacterium fatty acids and alcohol has been utilized for rapid and reliable identification of mycobacterium tuberculosis and atypical mycobacterium.

Chapter eleven

New Tools for Tuberculosis

SS Arora

Tuberculosis continues to be a public health problem, even in the 21st century. The WHO indicates that 1/3rd of the world population is infected with bacteria of mycobacterium tuberculosis complex, the causative agent of tuberculosis. This disease kills 2 and 3 million people worldwide annually. The emergence of drug resistance, especially multiple drug resistance, and increasing coinfection with HIV has further compounded the mortality. Early diagnosis of tuberculosis and drug resistance improves survival and by identifying infectious cases promotes contact tracing, implementation of institutional cross infection procedures, and other public health actions.

The conventional diagnostic methods of TB are microscopy and culture based on the methods first employed by Robert Koch who identified the cause of TB in 1882. Although sputum smear microscopy remains a cornerstone of tuberculosis control and is simple to perform, it has limited specificity and requires 10,000 to 1,00,000 organisms/ml and many cases of active TB may be missed using this method along. Fluorescent-staining methods possibly offer greater sensitivity.[1] Histopathology is characteristic but there could be problems to get representative specimen, and non-specific features. Traditional culture techniques are slow and can take many weeks to provide results causing delay in diagnosis and treatment. Immunology is often not conclusive as antibodies and delayed type hypersensitivity response persist for a long time after the subsidence of sub-clinical or clinical disease.

Modern Systems of Rapid Automated Liquid Cultures

Accurate diagnosis of tuberculosis is the identification of mycobacterium tuberculosis through culture, but the time required and the frequent negative results in paucibacillary specimens are important limitations.

Traditionally, culture has been grown on solid and liquid media such as Löwenstein-Jenson, or Kirchner and the various Middlebrook formulations. The time to detection of growth of a mycobacterial species can be shortened significantly with the use of an automated or semi-automated liquid culture system. Radiometric liquid culture using a broth with radiolabelled ^{14}C-palminate as its sole carbon source has been available for years.[2]

New fully automated systems that rely on non-radiometric detection of growth have been developed such as the MB/BacT, BACTEC 9000, and the Mycobacterial Growth Indicator Tube (MGIT). These systems measure changes in gas pressure, carbon dioxide production, oxygen consumption either florimetrically or colorimetrically. These systems need no further operator input (after loading) until the system signals positive. The importance of skilled and experienced staff cannot be overemphasized. Contamination rates have been high when inexperienced and untrained staff have used these systems.

Identification of Cultures

The genus mycobacterium includes M. tuberculosis complex which can cause tuberculosis in human beings, and environmental and opportunistic pathogens. Non-tuberculous-mycobacteira (NTM) usually cause disease in certain groups, particularly the immunocompromised. Rapid identification of M. tuberculosis complex can avoid unnecessary isolation of patients with NTM and implementation of costly and toxic treatment regimens.

1. Hybridization with specific gene probes.
2. Chemical analysis of lipid profiles, and
3. PCR methods, in combination with rapid culture has greatly reduced overall turnaround times for mycobacteriology laboratories.

Probe detection methods targeting ribosomal RNA, can identify M. tuberculosis complex, M. avium, M. intracellulare, M. avium complex, M. gordone and M. kansasii. These methods are rapid and simple, giving results in 1-2 hours with accuracy estimated to be above 90%, but cover a limited range of species.[3]

Mycobacteria have characteristic lipid profiles which can be analysed by HPLC.[4]

Commercially available rapid identification tests use PCR followed by reverse hybridization to identify the most clinically significant mycobacteria.[5] The system proved reliable in routine evaluations with 100% sensitivity from cultures and greater than 99% specificity, but the cost of these kits in routine use in prohibitive.

PCR restriction enzyme analysis of the *hsp65* gene is a more complex technique, but is more economical, flexible, and can identify mycobacteria from culture in 1-2 days.[6,7] Sequencing of the 165 rRNA gene allows rapid identification, but is relatively labour intensive and is best suited to the reference laboratory.

Phenotypic Detection

PCR based detection assays are not suitable for laboratories with poor resources. Alternative phenotypic assays based on mycobacteriophages have been developed. The incorporation of the *lux* gene, which codes for luciferase, into the phage allows detection of mycobacteriophage through emission of light and thus indirectly allows detection of viable M. tuberculosis. An alternative for detection of replicating phage involves the manual plating of phage onto a lawn of the rapidly growing host *Mycobacterium smegmatis*. Plates can be read visually by enumeration of clear areas of plaques on the lawn. This technology can also be applied to susceptibility testing of M. tuberculosis.

The newer methods for detection of growth of M. tuberculosis along with gene probe and gene amplification technologies have provided tools for rapid identification of isolates, direct detection of mycobacterial pathogens from clinical specimens and detection of drug resistance. Early diagnosis is of value clinically, and through the early institution of appropriate drug therapy is of public health benefit.

REFERENCES

1. Vestal AL. *Procedures for isolation and identification of mycobacteria,* US Department of Health, Education and Welfare Publication, NO, CDC 77-8230, CDC Atlanta, 1977.
2. Heifets LB, Good RB. Current laboratory methods for the diagnosis of tuberculosis. Washington: American Society for Microbiology, 1994:85-110.
3. Lebrun L, Espinasse F, Poveda JD *et al.* Evaluation of non-radioactive DNA probes for identification of mycobacteria. *J Clin Microbiol* 1992;30:2476-78.
4. Duffey PS *et al.* Improved rapid identification of mycobacteria by combining solid phase extraction with high performance liquid chromatographic (HPLC) analysis of BACTEC cultures. *J Clin Microbiol* 1996;34:1939-43.
5. Suffys PN, Silva Rocha A da *et al.* Rapid identification of Mycobacteria to species level using INNO-LiPA Mycobacteria, a reverse hybridization assay *J Clin Microbiol* 2001;39:4477-82.
6. Telenti A, Marchesi F *et al.* Rapid identification of mycobacteria to the species level by polymerase chain reaction and restriction enzyme analysis. *J Clin Microbiol* 1993;31:175-78.
7. Devallois A, Goh KS, *et al.* Rapid identification of mycobacteria to species level by PCR-restriction fragment length polymorphism analysis of the hsp65 gene and proposition of an algorithm to differentiate 34 mycobacterial species. *J Clin Microbiol* 1997;35:1079-84.

Chapter twelve

Pathological Diagnosis in Tubercular Lymphadenopathy

Kanchan Bhardwaj

Tuberculosis lymphadenitis is very common. Cervical group of lymphnodes are most commonly involved. The histopathological examination of the excised lymphnode is the most dependable diagnostic tool.[1] The definitive diagnosis is established by visualizing mycobacteria on histopathology sections. The AFB is demonstrated in 33.3% to 45.6% cases by ZN staining.[1-4] There is increase in percentage of AFB is seen in caseation necrosis (47%) with infiltration of polymorphs.[5-8] Conversely with more epithelioid cell granulomas, the percentage of AFB positivity declined (15%) as they limit the proliferation of AFB.[1,3] AFB culture positivity was reported in 16%-68% cases. For transportation of excised lymphnode selective Kirchner's liquid medium is best and specimens can be stored for upto 15 days without any loss in culture positivity.[9] As AFB is not demonstrated in many cases, certain other changes have been accepted as suggested of tuberculosis. These changes are not specific and may sometimes seen in other diseases also. These are granulomatous inflammation with caseation necrosis. However histopathological examination is time consuming, costly, requiring surgeon and anesthetist, and is associated with certain morbidity.[1]

Fine needle aspiration cytology (FNAC) is a simple, reliable, time conserving, out patient, economic technique having practically no complication and has a high patient acceptance. FNAC of the lymphnode is highly diagnostic (84.4%).[3] It has been suggested as the first diagnostic technique for the diagnosis of peripheral lymphadenopathy. The characteristic cytological features include epithelioid cell granulomas with or without multinucleated giant cells and caseation necrosis.[5,6,10-12] In a study on tubercular lymphadenitis these features are seen in decreasing frequency with epithelioid granulomas with caseation in 40.74% with AFB positivity in 7% and caseation necrosis only 10% with AFB positivity in 8% cases.[2] The sensitivity and specificity of FNAC of the tubercular lymphadenopathy is 77% and 93% respectively. FNAC proven tubercular lymphadenitis showed mycobacterial culture positivity in 49% and AFB was present in 30% of the direct and concentrated smears.[5] True positive diagnosis is reported in 83% cases, false negative in 24% and equivocal in 3% cases.

FNAC is a quick, reliable, inexpensive procedure with high diagnostic accuracy. However positive diagnosis is of value but a negative result may be noncontributory. If the clinical suspicion is strong, FNAC should be followed by lymphnode biopsy for histopathological examination.[1]

REFERENCES

1. Bhardwaj K, Bhardwaj BL, Goyal T. Fine needle aspiration cytology in lymphnode disorders with special reference to tuberculosis. J of cytology 2000; 17(3):155-59.
2. Das DK, Pant JM, Chachra KL. Tuberculous lymphadenitis, correlation of cellular components and necrosis in the lymphnode aspirates with AFB positivity and bacillary count. Ind J Pathol Microbio. 1999;33:1-10.
3. Dasgupta A, Gosh RN, Podder AK *et al.* Fine needle aspiration cytology of cervical lymphadenopathy with special reference to tuberculosis. J Ind Med Assoc 1994;92:44-46.
4. Parshad R, Garg SK, Mukerji PK, Aggarwal PK. Role of fine needle aspiration cytology in the diagnosis of lymphadenopathy. Ind J Chest Dis Allied Sci. 1993;35:27-29.
5. Gupta SK, Chug CD, Shiek XA, al Rubah NA. Cytodiagnosis of tubercular lymphadenitis. A correlative study of microbiologic examination. Acta Cytol 1993;35:329-32.
6. Lau SK, Wei WI, Hsu C *et al.* Efficacy of fine needle aspiration cytology in the diagnosis of tuberculous lymphadenopathy. J Larygol Otol. 1990;104:24-27.
7. Radhika S, Gupta SK, Chakarvarti A, Rajwanshi A, Joshi K. Role of culture of mycobacteria in fine needle aspiration diagnosis of tuberculous lymphadenitis. Diagn Cytopathol 1989;5:260-62.
8. Pithie AD, Chicksen B. Fine needle extra thoracic lymphnode aspiration in HIV associated sputum negative tuberculosis. Lancet 1992;340:1504-05.
9. Vanajakumar, Selvakumar N, Jawahar MS *et al.* Transportation of lymphnode biopsy specimens in selective Kirchner's liquid medium for culture of tubercle bacilli. J Med Microbiol 1997;46:260-62.
10. Gupta AK, Nayer M, Chandra M. Critical appraisal of fine needle aspiration cytology in tuberculous lymphadenitis. Acta Cytologica 1992;36:391-94.
11. Finfer M, Perchik A, Burstein DE. Fine needle aspiration biopsy diagnosis of tuberculosis lymphadenitis in patients with or without immunodeficiency syndrome. Acta Cytol 1991:35:325-32.
12. Orell SR, Gregory FS, Walter MN-I, Witaker D. Lymphnode. In manual and atlas of fine needle aspiration cytology. Ed-Orell SR,Gregory FS, Walter MN-I, Witaker D. Churchill Livingstone 1992;63-94.

Chapter thirteen

Utility of Chest Imaging in Diagnosis of Pulmonary Tuberculosis

Amir M Khoja, Sandip Ghodekar, Mangesh M Dande

INTRODUCTION

In this chapter we will try to elaborate the role of conventional radiology of chest and that of advance modalities like HRCT, MRI, Ultrasonography, bronchial angiography and embolisation in the diagnosis and the management of tuberculosis.

There are different organs getting involved in the process of tuberculosis. These affections give different radiological pictures. These findings on radiology may not be gold standard but along with clinical and other pathological investigations become almost total diagnostic of tuberculosis.

Chest Wall Tuberculosis

Rib erosion along with localized swelling on the chest wall makes one suspect tuberculosis of chest wall. It is secondary to lung or hematogenous origin. Soft tissue mass in the chest wall with or without bony destruction is the radiographic findings of rib tuberculosis (Fig. 13.1)

Juxtacostal soft tissue mass with central low attenuation and peripheral rim enhancement is the CT findings of rib tuberculosis.[1] Bony destruction, osteolytic

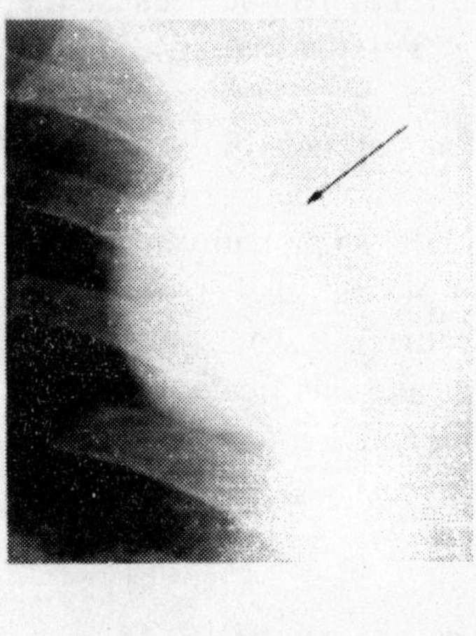

Fig. 13.1: X-rays chest showing soft tissue mass in the chest wall with bony destruction

expansile lesions with cortical disruption or mild cortical irregularity, may be associated. In addition to ribs, costal cartilage, sternoclavicular joint and thoracic spine can be involved with tuberculous process. In these cases, osseous and cartilaginous destruction, soft tissue mass with calcification, and rim enhancement of soft tissue mass following intravenous contrast medium administration are the CT findings.

MRI is occasionally helpful in evaluating the complication of tuberculosis, such as extent of thoracic wall involvement with empyema.

Pleural Tuberculosis

Pleural effusion probably occur in about 10% of all new tuberculous infection. The frequency is higher in adult patients with AIDS.[2]

On plain radiograph tubercular pleural effusion appears either as free fluid along the chest wall or loculated in lateral or mediastinal pleura (Fig. 13.2). Sometimes nodularity can be appreciated on pleural surface on the radiograph.[3]

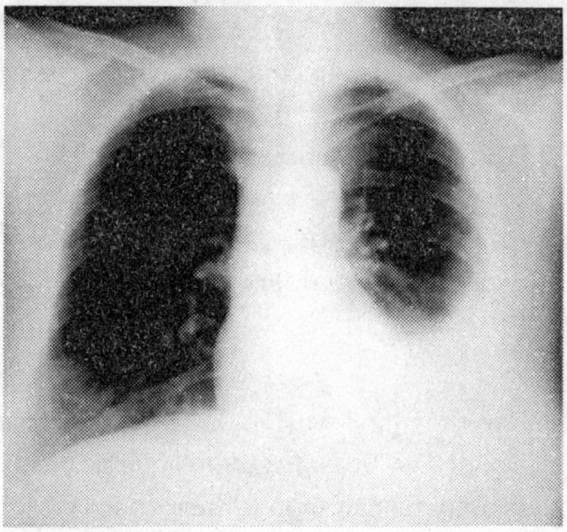

Fig. 13.2: X-ray showing pleural effusion along with chest wall

In early tuberculous effusion, ultrasonography may show simple anechoic pleural fluid. It is very sensitive test for the presence of fluid but not a very specific as far as the volume of fluid is concerned. This may be because the pleural space is three diamensional space with gross volume change in supine and sitting position.

In acute tuberculous effusion, CT scan may show parenchymal cavitation including small subpleural cavity, the site of communication between the cavity and the pleural space, parenchymal infiltrates, and hilar adenopathy as well as fluid collection in the pleural cavity. Thin, regular pleural thickening can be shown on CT scans. In chronic tuberculous empyema, CT scan shows focal fluid collection in association with pleural thickening and calcification. In these cases, the presence of residual pleural fluid signifies active infection.[4]

Empyema is visualized on contrast-enhanced CT scans with enhancement of the parietal and visceral pleurae. They may demonstrate enhancing septa within the pleural fluid collections. The pleural fluid collections are characterized by low attenuation; however, they do not have attenuation values consist with simple fiuid. Empyemas demonstrate the so-called split pleura sign. This sign consists of the pleural fluid collection tracking between the abnormally enhancing parietal and visceral pleura.

Spontaneous pneumothorax is an uncommon complication of disease, may be secondary to peripherally located lesions.

PARENCHYMAL TUBERCULOSIS

Primary Tuberculosis

Primary tuberculosis usually appears with lobar pneumonia combined with radiologically recognizable enlargement of lymph nodes in the hilum or the mediastinum (Fig. 13.3). Lobar pneumonia usually involves one lobe, however, two or more lobes may be involved.[2,5]

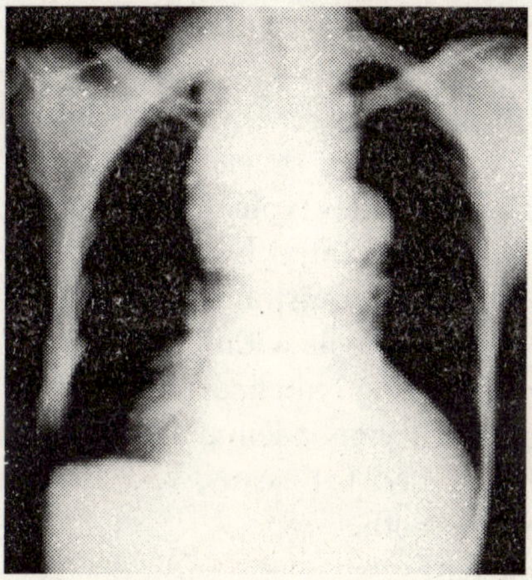

Fig. 13.3: X-ray showing right paratracheal lymphnodal mass

On radiograph and CT scans, the consolidation is usually homogeneous, dense, and well defined. It is anatomically confined to a segment, or more commonly a lobe. With progression especially in patients who are immunocompromised, have diabetes, or are taking corticosteroids, lobar or segmental pneumonia breaks down into a cavity. Primary tuberculosis appears as a solitary cavitary lesion in about 10% of patients (Fig. 13.4).[2]

Acute bronchogenic spread of tuberculosis occurs from breakdown of a lobar infection or from rupture of an infected lymph node into the bronchus. On radiographs, several foci of the lung are typically involved often remote from one another. Typical CT findings in bronchogenic spread of pulmonary tuberculosis are foci of nodular densities that vary markedly in size (larger

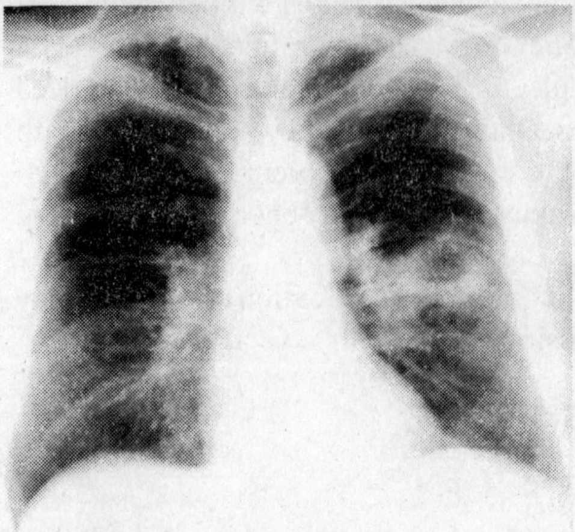

Fig. 13.4: Cavitatory lesion LLL

than those in miliary tuberculosis). The densities comprise combinations of centrilobular branching linear structure, relatively poorly defined centrilobular peribronchial nodules 2-3 mm in size, acinar shadows 4-10 mm in size, and large lobular consolidations.[2,6]

- CT helps confirm the presence of an ill-defined parenchymal infiltrate, as well as lymphadenopathy.
- CT scans may demonstrate enlarged lymph nodes typically measuring more than 2 cm. Lymph nodes demonstrate central hypoattenuation with peripheral rim enhancement with the administration of contrast material. This appearance reflects central necrosis within the node.
- CT is the examination of choice for evaluating lymphadenopathy and involvement of the tracheobronchial tree. Lymphadenopathy causing bronchial compression can be identified on CT scans, and airway compromise can be monitored during chemotherapy.
- Broncholiths may be identified in rare cases.
- Morphologically, the stenoses in active disease are areas of irregular luminal narrowing with circumferential wall thickening.

Postprimary Tuberculosis

Postprimary tuberculosis appears with local exudative lesions, local fibronodular lesions, cavitation, and bronchogenic spread of tuberculosis on radiographs. Cavitation is a particularly important manifestation of tuberculosis. Approximately 40% of adults with tuberculosis have some form of cavitation, usually in combination with pulmonary infiltration (Fig. 13.5).[7]

Im *et al.*[6] evaluated the HRCT findings of active pulmonary tuberculosis in 41 newly diagnosed patients. The findings were centrilobular lesions appearing as a nodule or branching linear structure (95%), bronchial wall thickening (73%),

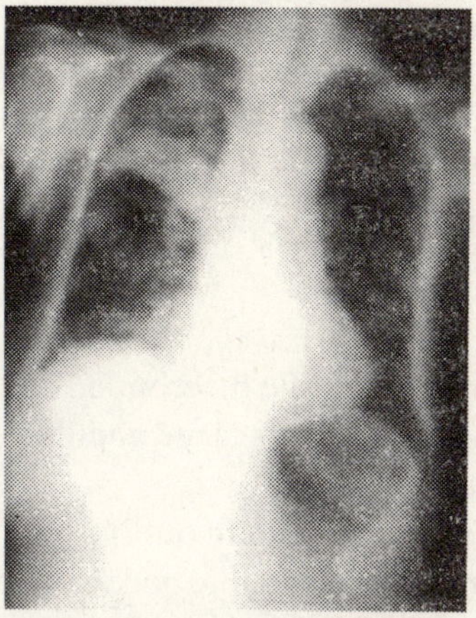

Fig. 13.5: X-ray chest showing parenchymal infiltrates RUL with cavitation

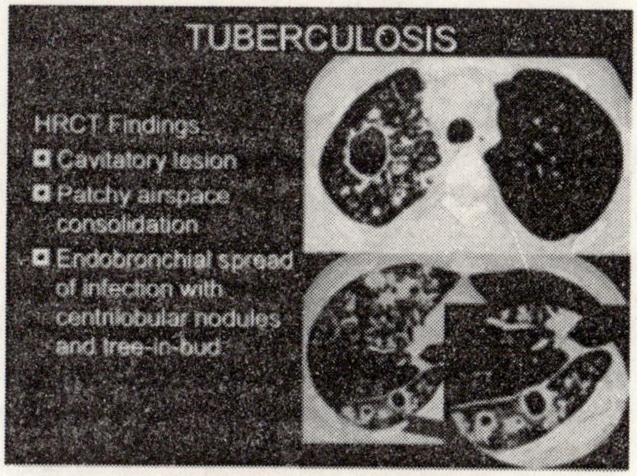

Fig. 13.6: HRCT showing cavitation and tree in bud appearance

tree-in-bud appearance (71%), poorly defined nodule (61%), cavity (51%), and lobular consolidation (41%) (Fig. 13.6).

Terminal tufts of the tree-in-bud represent lesions within the bronchioles and alveolar ducts, while the stalk represents a lesion in the last-order bronchus within the secondary lobule. Larger areas of consolidation on pathologic examination manifested the areas of lobular and lobar consolidation on CT scan. Lobular consolidation consisted of centrally located granulomas that contained caseation necrosis and marginal nonspecific inflammation; the area of inflammation appeared relatively loose compared with the central granuloma with caseation necrosis. On the other hand, the findings of inactive or stable state of pulmonary tuberculosis on HRCT scans included areas of irregular lines and calcified nodules along with distortion of bronchovascular bundles, bronchiectasis, and pericicatrical emphysema.[6]

In postprimary tuberculosis, CT accurately demonstrates the pattern, distribution, and extent of the parenchymal lesion. Cavities, the most important radiological evidence of activity, can be well depicted on CT. The nature of pulmonary damage, including bronchiectasis, cicatrization atelectasis and scarring, can be characterized. Furthermore CT is also useful in deciphering chest radiographs when extensive disease makes interpretation difficult.[8]

CT scans may be helpful in evaluating parenchymal involvement, satellite lesions, bronchogenic spread of infection, and miliary disease.

- Cavitation is best demonstrated on CT scans. The outer wall of the cavity tends to be thick walled and irregular, whereas the inner wall tends to be smooth. An air-fluid level may be identified. The connection of the cavity to the airway may be visualized. Complications of cavitary disease may become apparent with mycetoma formation, which appears as an intraluminal collection of material with a crescent of surrounding

air. Changes in patient positioning demonstrate a change in the position of the mycetoma relative to the cavity.
- The bronchogenic spread of tuberculosis is recognized on CT scans by the presence of acinar shadows and nodules of varying sizes in a peribronchial distribution. The lesions are seen throughout both lungs.

Tuberculoma

Primary tuberculosis in adults may appear as solitary or multiple macronodular lesions (tuberculomas).[5] Postprimary tuberculosis also presents large nodular or mass-like densities that are considered neoplastic.

The tuberculomas on CT scans are usually regular and smooth in outline but may have a rough edge. Cavitation in the lesion or surrounding satellite nodule(s), sometimes enabling differentiation from lung cancer on CT scans, can be seen on CT scans. The lesions are usually low in attenuation and show no. of minimal enhancement with contrast medium administration. Calcification in the tuberculomas is found in 20-30% of the lesions and is usually nodular and diffuse.[9] Rarely tuberculoma appears with CT-halo sign (halo of round-glass attenuation surrounding the nodule) in a patient with hemoptysis.[10]

Miliary Tuberculosis

In the early stage of miliary tuberculosis, chest radiography may appear normal. Follow-up radiography obtained a week or more later usually shows a poorly defined haze through both lungs. Typical nodules of 1-2 mm become recognizable even as late as 2-3 months (Fig. 13.7). As the infection progresses, the miliary nodules coalesce. Cavitation may occasionally occur in the nodules.[5]

HRCT scans show poorly or well-defined, well marginated nodules of 1-2 mm in size widely disseminated throughout the lungs in association with diffuse reticulation (Fig. 13.8). Other features attributable to the presence of nodules included nodular interlobular septae, nodular irregularity of vessels, subpleural

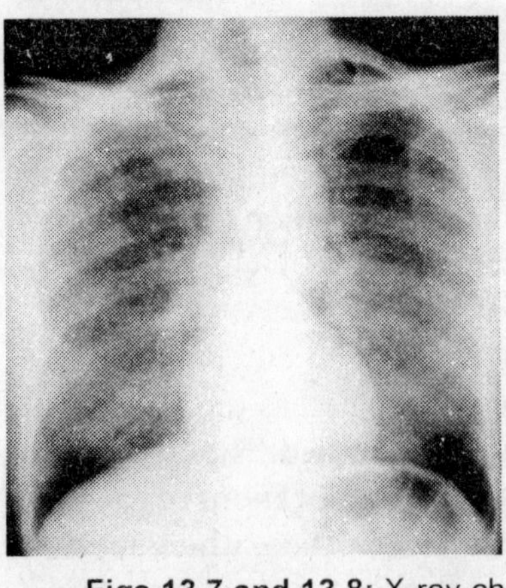

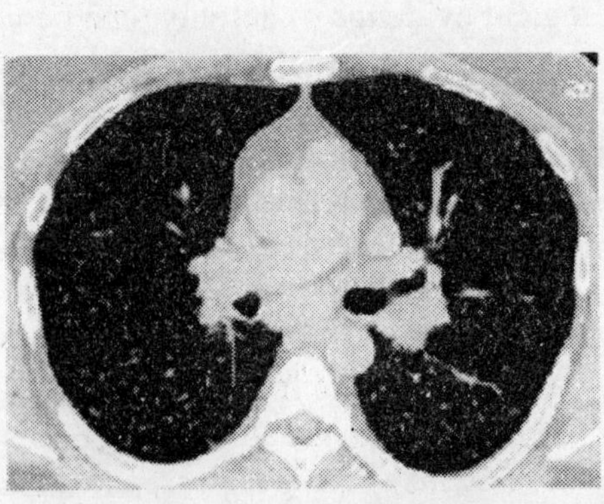

Figs 13.7 and 13.8: X-ray chest and HRCT showing miliary tuberculosis

dots and studded fissures. Diffuse intra- and interlobular septal thickening are also common.[11]

The role of CT scan in the diagnosis of miliary tuberculosis is in the conditions when the patient is ill, particularly in a fever of unknown origin, and chest radiograph is normal. In this condition, HRCT may show ill-defined nodules that were not definite on chest radiograph, rendering transbronchial lung biopsy for the diagnosis of miliary lung disease.

CT scans may aid in the evaluation of uncommon complications of miliary tuberculosis, e.g., adult respiratory distress syndrome (ARDS) and pulmonary hemorrhage resulting from disseminated intravascular coagulopathy. Both ARDS and pulmonary hemorrhage may manifest as alveolar filling in a background of miliary nodules.

Airway Tuberculosis

Airway involvement in tuberculosis has been reported in 10-20% of all patients with pulmonary tuberculosis.[12] The airways can be involved secondarily by the spreads of organism within the airway lumen or along peribronchial lymphatic channels from an area of cavitation or localized tuberculous pneumonia. They can also be involved by direct extension of infection from a contiguous lymph node or parenchyma itself.[13]

Usually airway tuberculosis presents with persistent infiltration, atelectasis, cavitating lesion, mass-like lesion or rarely miliary mottling on plain radiograph. On CT scans the involved bronchi shows stenosis with wall thickening, obstruction with peribronchial cuff of soft tissue, stenosis or obstruction with adjacent tuberculous lymphadenitis or intraluminal polypoid mass of low attenuation with bronchial narrowing.[12]

Bronchiectasis is a well-known sequela of postprimary disease (Fig. 13.9). Bronchiectasis tends to occur in the upper lobes and often manifests as traction bronchiectasis on the basis of fibrotic disease with subsequent traction on the airways. Recurrent infections and hemoptysis may result from traction bronchiectasis.

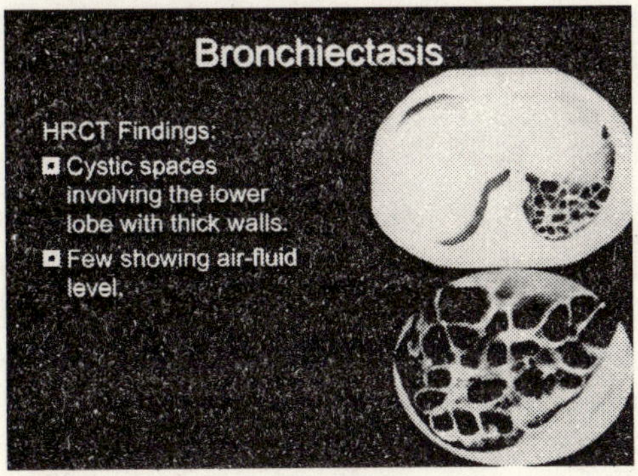

Fig. 13.9: HRCT showing cystic bronchiectasis

The role of CT in the evaluation of airway tuberculosis is to explain the mechanism of airway involvement by showing the bronchial lesion per se or surrounding enlarged lymph nodes in the mediastinum or the hilum. Another role of CT in the bronchial tuberculosis is its usefulness in the follow-up of the response to treatment, especially when the bronchial biopsy shows only nonspecific or indeterminate results.

Bronchial tuberculosis may cause diagnostic problem with overlapping features with bronchogenic carcinoma both on radiographs and CT scans. Minimal and uniform thickening of the bronchial wall in tuberculous bronchitis may simulate the finding of early bronchogenic carcinoma. The presence of enlarged lymph nodes lying close to the stenotic bronchus with low attenuation on enhanced CT scans, when combined with peripheral parenchymal atelectasis or consolidation, may mimic the findings of lung cancer showing differential enhancement between a central tumor mass and atelectatic distal lung. Because of these overlapping features between bronchial tuberculosis and bronchogenic carcinoma, bronchoscopy should be performed to confirm the diagnosis.

Mediastinal Tuberculosis

Tuberculous lymphadenitis often with an associated pulmonary lesion (the primary complex) is a frequent manifestation of primary tuberculosis in children. The lesion is not uncommon in adults. The radiographic finding varied, however, very often includes right tracheobronchial involvement.

On enhancement CT scans, nodes larger than 2 cm in diameter invariably shows central areas of low attenuation and peripheral rim enhancement. Enhanced walls are usually irregular in thickness. In a small number of patients, solid or calcified type of nodes could be observed.[14]

On MR, tuberculous lymphadenitis with central areas of flow attenuation and peripheral rim enhancement at CT sans shows homogenous nodes with hyperintensity both on T1 and T2 weighted images. The lymphadenitis with solid type at CT scans similarly shows homogenous nodes with hyperintensity on both T1 and T2 weighted images but less marked T2 prolongation than that with central areas of low attenuation and peripheral rim enhancement. The lymphadenitis with calcification shows in homogenous nodes with hypointensity both on T1 and T2 weighted images.[15]

Pericardial Tuberculosis

Pericardial disease can be imaged with CT or MRI, although calcification related to prior tuberculous pericarditis is more readily apparent on CT images.

Typically, ultrasonography is not useful in imaging pulmonary disease. Ultrasonography may be used for thoracentesis guidance or to evaluate the pericardium for secondary tuberculous involvement.

Role of Nuclear Medicine in Tuberculosis

There is no definitive role of nuclear medicine in the diagnosis of tuberculosis.

Bronchography

Bronchography very clearly demonstrates the tracheobronchial lesions though hardly performed these days because of unavailability of the dye.

Role of Interventional Radiology in Tuberculosis

Interventional radiologic techniques may be used to confirm the diagnosis of tuberculosis with percutaneous lymph node aspiration or biopsy to obtain material for culture, cytologic, or histologic studies. Biopsy can be taken either under fluoroscopic control or CT guided or ultrasonography guided.

Stent placement or bronchoplasty can be done for the patients of post tubercular bronchostenosis under fluoroscopy guidance by bronchoscopist.

Angiography is not used in the diagnosis of pulmonary tuberculosis. Angiographic techniques such as bronchial arteriography and embolization in patients with hemoptysis may be used to treat the complications of pulmonary tuberculosis where dilated tortuous arteries can cause bleeding (Fig. 13.10). Excellent results are obtained with the embolisation with Gel foam and coils (Fig. 13.11). The changes in the anatomy of the origin of the bronchial arteries must be thought of in the patients with lot of fibrotic lesions and bronchiectasis due to tuberculosis. Considering the bilateral nature of the disease and inoperability makes bronchial artery embolisation a procedure of choice in moderate to severe hemoptysis.[16]

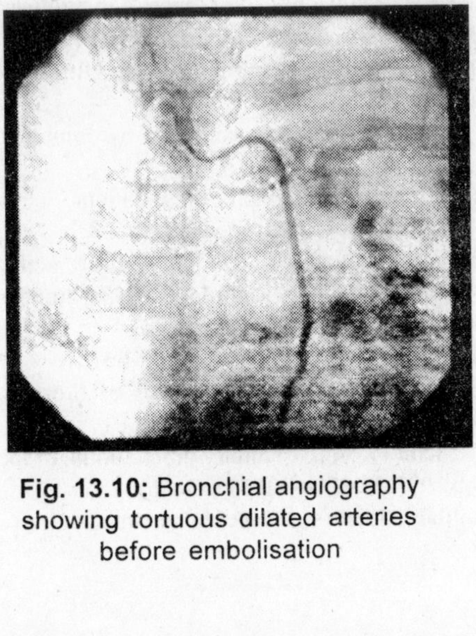

Fig. 13.10: Bronchial angiography showing tortuous dilated arteries before embolisation

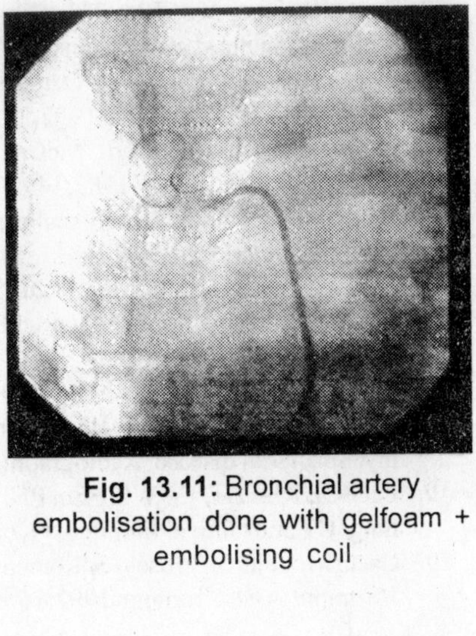

Fig. 13.11: Bronchial artery embolisation done with gelfoam + embolising coil

SUMMARY

The chest X-ray is indicated in persons suspected of having TB who are sputum smear-negative and who do not respond to 2 weeks of antibiotic therapy. No radiographic pattern in pathognomonic of TB, although the classical hallmarks of the disease are cavitation, apical distribution, pulmonary fibrosis, shrinkage and calcification. HIV infected persons with a well preserved immune function will show these typical features. However, as immune suppression worsens, chest X-rays more often show atypical findings such as pulmonary infiltrates affecting the lower lobes, intrathoracic lymphadenopathy miliary tuberculosis and rarely a normal chest radiograph. Disease other than TB can cause both the classical and atypical chest X-ray findings, and if sputum smears are negative, other conditions have to be considered in the differential diagnosis.

Conventional radiography plays a important role in the diagnosis of pulmonary tuberculosis and pathological changes in the air content of the lungs. Bronchography is now rarely used for the demonstration of fine changes in the bronchial tree. CT is very useful mode of examination for the visualization of the features of pulmonary changes and localized lesions in pulmonary tuberculosis. MR is of less importance; it possibly plays a role in examinations of the mediastinal lesions. The bronchial and definite role in the treatment of hemoptysis due to tuberculosis.

To conclude chest imaging is a most important tool in the diagnosis of tuberculosis along with the clinical and pathological correlation.

REFERENCES

1. Lee G. Im J-G, Kim JS, Kang HS, Han MC. Tuberculosis of the ribs: CT appearance. J Comput Assist Tomogr 1993;17:363-366.
2. Lee KS, Song KS, Lim TH, Kim PN, Lee BH. Adult onset pulmonary tuberculosis: Findings on chest radiographs and CT scans.
3. Akhan O. Demirkazik FB, Ozmen MN, *et al.* Tuberculous pleural effusion: Ultrasonic diagnosis Clin Ultrasound 1992;20:461-465.
4. Hulnick DH, Niaidch DP, McCauley DI. Pleural tuberculosis evaluated by computed tomography Radiology 1983;149:759-765.
5. Palmer PES. Pulmonary tuberculosis: Usual and unusual radiographic presentations. Semin Roentgenol 1979;14:204-243.
6. Im J-G, Itoh H. Shim Y-S, *et al.* Pulmonary tuberculosis: CT findings—Early active disease and sequential change with antituberculous therapy. Radiology 1993;186:653-660.
7. Miller WT. Tuberculosis in the 1990s. Radiol Clin North Am 1994;32:649-661.
8. Kuhiman TE, Deutsch JH, Fishman EK, Siegelman SS. CT features of thoracic mycobacterial disease. Radiographics 1990;14:413-431.
9. Lee KS, Kim HT, Co WS, Kim PN, Bae WK, Kim IY. Active solitary tuberculoma of the lung: CT and clinical findings. J Kor Rad Soc 1993;29:1200-1207 (Korean).
10. Gaeta M, Volta S. Stroscio S. Romeo P, Pandolfo I. CT halo sign in pulmonary tuberculoma. J Comput Assist Tomogr 1992;16:827-828.

11. McGuiness G. Naidich DP, Jagirdar J. Leitmen B. McCauley DI. High resolution CT findings in miliary lung disease. J Comput Assist Tomogr 1992;16:384-390.
12. Lee KS, Kim YH, Kim WS, Hwang SH, Kim PN, Lee BH. Endobronchial tuberculosis: CT features J Comput Assist Tomogr 1991;15:424-428.
13. Ip MSM, So SY, Lam WK, Mok CK. Endobronchial tuberculosis revisited. Chest 1986;89:727-73.
14. Im J-G, Song KS, Kang HS, *et al.* Mediastinal tuberculous lymphadenitis: CT manifestations. Radiology 1987;164:115-119.
15. Moon WK, Im J-G, Han MC. CT and MR imaging of mediastinal tuberculous lymphadenitis. Radiology 1993;189 (p):437.
16. Khoja Amir M. Bronchial Artery Embolization: Life saving therapy for hemoptysis. Journal of Bronchology. January 2003;10(1):22-29.

Chapter fourteen

Role of Fibre-optic Bronchoscopy in the Diagnosis of Pulmonary Tuberculosis

P Bhattacharya, Abhijit Mukerjee

Fibre-optic bronchoscopy has been a recent and effective arm in the armamentarium for diagnosis of pulmonary tuberculosis. Conventionally, the diagnosis of pulmonary tuberculosis has been limited to sputum examination for AFB by smear and culture. They are not universally positive and although the specificity is very high, the sensitivities vary widely depending on several factors. Which are often beyond the control of the investigator.

Tubercular lesions of the lungs are of varied nature morphologically and pathologically. Confirmed diagnosis is essential from the viewpoint of treatment since not only the cause of the disease is important for the sufferer and the society, a wrong diagnosis may often lead to undesired consequences since tuberculosis can mimic many other diseases of lungs including malignancy.

Fibre-optic bronchoscopy happens to be a relatively non-invasive tool to examine the tracheobronchial tree; it has traversed a long way from its 1st use by Ikeda.[1] Apart from visualization of the tracheobronchial tree, sampling of the airway secretion, lavage of the distal airways and alveoli and making transbronchial biopsy of diseased lung parenchyma have been successful through FOB. Authors have done bronchial aspiration, bronchial washing, bronchial brushing, bronchial biopsy, bronchoalveolar lavage, transbronchial lung biopsy, transbronchial needle aspiration and like procedure to collect samples to perform histological, microbiological (ZN staining and AFB culture) and molecular studies (PCR for mycobacterial DNA identification) to identify and confirm tubercular lesions. In addition, it has been found that post bronchoscopic sputum has got higher yield for both smear and culture examinations.

Indication of Bronchoscopy in Tuberculosis

1. Smear negative cases with high index of suspicion for tuberculosis.

2. Patients/subjects who cannot cough or can cough without expectoration with high index of suspicion for pulmonary tuberculosis.
3. In case of confusion with other pathologies in clinico-radiologically suggestive or even sputum positive tuberculosis.
4. Selected patients with even sputum culture negativity for AFB with high index of suspicion.
5. In cases of suspected atypical mycobacterial infection (MAC) as evident from HRCT findings.

The Procedure of Bronchoscopy for Tuberculosis

1. The performer should take all precautions to avoid the contamination of the disease to him and the other HCWs.
2. Contamination of the scope and proper disinfection to prevention spread of the disease through procedure.

Different Bronchoscopic Procedures and Yields

Bronchoscopic samples can give an early diagnosis from detection of mycobacteria in smear or granuloma in biopsy. However, AFB culture of the collected samples takes a few weeks to give an answer.

Smear examination of the bronchial washing, bronchial aspirate, bronchoalveolar lavage, and TBLB can give early diagnosis of tuberculosis.[2] Bronchial washing has a better yield in both smear and culture examination compared to bronchial aspirate.[2] It appears that BAL has got very high yield compared to washing and brushing samples.[3] The yield of TBLB for the diagnosis of tuberculosis is variable from 7.5 to 75 percent in sputum smear negative tuberculosis.[2,4] In addition, TBLB has a role in excluding tuberculosis in a suspected non-tubercular disease[4,5] and also in confirming the atypical presentation of a non-tuberculous disease (especially malignancy) in an initially suspected tubercular lesion.[4-6] Considering all these, TBLB may be recommended in all bronchoscopies with parenchymal lesions having sputum smear negativity.[4]

Post-bronchoscopic sputum has also got a much higher yield in initial sputum negative tuberculosis from smear examination but not from culture.[2] Brushing smears for AFB was found useful especially when done from areas of affection and caseation.[7]

Bronchoalveolar lavage is positive in about 25 and 50 percent respectively in smear and culture in sputum smear negative tuberculosis.[8] Bronchial mucosal biopsy from suspected cases of endobronchial tuberculosis is helpful.[8] transbronchial needle aspiration is also worthwhile at times.[8]

It has been found that combining one, two, three or more procedures increases the overall diagnostic probability. However, it is observed that TBLB culture does not add much to the diagnostic yield.[8]

Bronchoscopy in Atypical Mycobacterial Infection

Bronchoscopy has been found to be helpful in diagnosis of radiologically suspected MAC infection in smear negative cases[9] where the smear and culture positivity of bronchial washing goes to as high as 44 and 85 percent respectively, while TBLB appears much less efficient.[9] FOB can help to differentiate infection from colonization in MAC infection. It should be sought in cases where HRCT shows nodular opacities around ecstatic bronchi.[9] In a retrospective analysis, 31.25% of the diagnosis of culture positive tuberculosis were done solely from bronchoscopic samples;[5] the yield of bronchoscopic samples were comparable to the yield of sputum culture.[5]

Value of PCR in Bronchoscopic Samples

PCR being highly sensitive (97.2%) for identification of the DNA of mycobacteria in bronchoscopic samples has also got a high negative predictive value (95.2%). Hence, it is no way superior to the conventional tests of smear or culture examinations and may be of just ancillary value in the diagnosis of the smear negative cases.[10]

Bronchoscopy in HIV Positive Tuberculosis Patients

Smear and culture positive of bronchoscopic samples are comparable in regards of diagnostic yields for tuberculosis with or without HIV co-infection. However, the yield of TBLB is less (< 50%) in TB-HIV patients.[11]

Can FOB Lead to Tuberculosis?

Yes, a contaminated bronchoscope can spread tubercular and atypical myobacterial infection1[12,13] or even MDR tuberculosis.[14] Hence proper sterilization of the scope is essential before use.[15,16]

REFERENCES

1. Ikeda S, Yanni N, Ishikawa S: Flexible bronchofiberscope, Keio J Med 1968;17:1-16.
2. Kekkaku. Diagnostic value of bronchoscopy in diagnosis of pulmonary tuberculosis: Bronchial aspirate, bronchial washing and transbronchial lung biopsy 1990 Jan; 65(1):33-36.
3. J de Gracia, V Curull, R. Vidal, A Riba, R Orriols, N Martin and F Morell. Diagnostic value of bronchoalveolar lavage in suspected pulmonary tuberculosis. Chest Vol 93;329-332.
4. Charoenratanakul S, Dejsomritrutai W, Chaiprasert A. Diagnostic role of fibreoptic bronchoscopy in suspected smear negative pulmonary tuberculosis. Respir Med 1995 Oct 89(9):621-23.
5. Wong CF, Yew WW, Chan CY, Au LY, Cheung SW, Cheng AF. Rapid diagnosis of smear-negative pulmonary tuberculosis via fibreoptic bronchoscopy: Utility of polymerase chain reaction in bronchial aspirates as an adjunct to transbronchial biopsies. Respir Med 1998;92(6):815-19.

6. Jayasundera CI, Attapattu M, Kumarasinghe MP. Atypical presentations of pulmonary tuberculosis diagnosed by fibreoptic bronchoscopy. Postgrad Med J. 1993 Aug;69(814):621-23.
7. Chawla R, Pant K, Jaggi OP, Chandrashekhar S, Thukral SS. Fibreoptic bronchoscopy in smear-negative pulmonary tuberculosis. Eur Respir J 1998 Oct;1(9):804-06.
8. Yuksekol I, Bal S, Ozkan M, Balkan A, Bedirhan I, Tozkoparan E, Demirci N, Seber O. The value of fibreoptic bronchoscopy in diagnosis of smear negative pulmonary tuberculosis. Tiberk Toraks 2003;51(4):405-09.
9. Ikedo Y. Kurume Med J 2001;48(1):15-19. The significance of bronchoscopy for the diagnosis of mycobacterium avium complex (MAC) pulmonary disease.
10. Kennedy DJ, Lewis WP, Barnes PF. Yield of bronchoscopy for the diagnosis of tuberculosis in patients with human immunodeficiency virus infection. Chest 1992 Oct;102(4):1040-44.
11. Mehta J, Krish G, Berro E, Harvill L. Fibreoptic bronchoscopy in the diagnosis of pulmonary tuberculosis. BMJ 2000;321:465-466 (19 August).
12. Wheeler PW, Lancaster D, Kaiter AB; Bronchopulmoanry cross-colonization and infection related to mycobacterial contamination of suction valves of bronchoscope; J. Infect Dis 1989;159:954-58.
13. Prigogine T *et al.*; Mycobacterial cross-contamination of bronchoscopy specimens; J Hosp Infect; 1988;11:93-95.
14. Agaton T *et al.*; Transmission of a highly drug-resistant strain (strain W) of mycobacterium tuberculosis; JAMA; 1997;278;1073-77.
15. Hamson PJV *et al.*; A study of glutaraldehyde disinfection of fibreoptic bronchoscope experimentally contaminated mycobacterium tuberculosis J.Hosp Infect; 1992;22:137-42.
16. Seballos RL, Walsh AL, Mehta AC; Clinical evaluation and liquid chemical sterilization system for flexible bronchoscope; J. Bronchol; 1995;2:192-99.

Chapter fifteen

Management of Pulmonary TB

RS Bhatia

INTRODUCTION

Pulmonary tuberculosis, a product of combination of socio-economic as well as biological factors,[1] is very much in the reach of clinician with the adequate diagnosing methods and the widely accepted short course chemotherapy.[2] But the problem of containing and eradicating this disease stands unsolved even to date. One suffers from pulmonary tuberculosis if he secretes tubercle bacilli in the sputum and rest in whom the disease is not confirmed bacteriologically are called 'suspect cases' as is defined by WHO. Perhaps, these cases are to be followed up, rather than giving them drug treatment.[3]

Pathogenesis

Pathogenesis includes destruction of polymorphonuclear cells by the tubercle bacillus followed by ingestion, at the beginning of infection. Here it multiplies slowly but regularly in the macrophage, one of which drains to the respective lymph nodes, thus presenting tubercle bacillus antigen to T lymphocytes. Specifically responsive clones of T cells get activated and replicated and get poured in large numbers into the blood circulation, giving rise to tuberculin hypersensitivity (T-cell reaction to tuberculoprotein) and tuberculoimmunity (T-cell reactive to immunizing antigen). The hypersensitive T-cells are probably destructive ones, causing tissue damage, leading to tubercle formation and producing growth enhancing factor (GEF), while immune T-cells chiefly induce tuberculocidal macrophages. The immune T lymphocytes evoke release of lymphokines called growth inhibition factor (GIF), which activate the arriving macrophages in such a manner that destroy the tubercle bacilli that they ingest. The bacilli are easily killed if they are multiplying. But once they stop multiplication, they get spared and thus called dormant bacilli.

When cell mediated immunity fails, a pathogenic GEF-producing response takes up the charge, the activated macrophages die, releasing proteolytic enzymes in the lung tissue, which in turn destroy the tissue causing caseous necrosis and cavitation.[2] The pathogenesis clearly creates a demand for antitubercular drugs to be bactericidal, effective at killing the organisms both at extracellular as well as intracellular level in the overall management of pulmonary Koch's infection.

Drugs and Mechanism of Drug Action

Most of the antitubercular drugs are bactericidal (bacteriostatic drugs being thiacetazone and PAS), the isoniazid being the most potent.[4,5] It has been estimated that isoniazid alone may kill some 90% of bacillary population during the first few days of chemotherapy.[5] And in drug combination regimen, isoniazid again scores the highest bactericidal activity.[2]

Isoniazid and rifampicin have a strong bactericidal action against continuously and relatively rapidly multiplying organisms, but the pyrazinamide is most effective against slowly multiplying tubercle bacilli within the macrophages. Rifampicin has a unique sterilizing action, killing dormant bacilli or persisters within hours of their starting multiplying. And pyrazinamide kills a special population of bacteria in an acid environment inside the macrophages while streptomycin has poor penetration capability into the cells, the ethambutol blocks the ability of tubercle bacilli to build and maintain their cells wall, thus killing them by attrition rather than by direct action.

And there exists still another group—the dormant group of tubercle bacilli which are not killed by any of the drugs. To sum up, isoniazid and rifampicin are bactericidal, important bactericidal being the rifampicin; the streptomycin and pyrazinamide are less potent bactericidal rifampicin and pyrazinamide being most important sterilizing agents, capable of killing semi-dormant bacilli which has ability to survive the bactericidal action of isoniazid and so giving rise to relapse. Ethambutol is bactericidal, although the difference between adequate therapeutic and toxic dose becomes sometimes small. Isoniazid and rifampicin take the lead in preventing the emergence of drug resistance. All drugs are effective both in intermittent and daily dose regimen except for thiacetazone which is less effective when given intermittently.[2,4,5]

Apart from streptomycin, ethambutol, pyrazinamide, isoniazid and rifampicin (which are commonly used in definite three or more drug regimens), reserve drugs include ethionamide, cycloserine, thiacetazone, capreomycin, PAS, kanamycin and viomycin. Newer drugs under experimental stages are amikacin, cyclorifamycin, slow release depot injection and immunotherapeutic agents.[2]

Diagnosis

Before we go for treatment, it is the diagnosis which is important. Chest skiagram and tuberculin testing are very good aids but never conclusive. Chest X-ray is never typical one for pulmonary Kochs since many pulmonary diseases simulate in radiographic findings. Over added is the observer's error to the tune of 25%.[2] Mantoux testing, done by injecting 0.1 ml solution, intradermally of 5 TU PPD on forearm and reaching after 72 hours, results an induration which if it is more than 10 mm in the transverse plane is usually considered positive. Serological tests include SAFA, ELISA, DATE and LPT but significant number of culture positive patients do not manifest circulating antibodies and the disease remission is not essentially followed by a decrease in antibody level.[2]

The bactec system using a culture substrate labelled with C^{14} (which is metabolized to radioactive carbon dioxide gas) helps getting very rapid culture growth of bacteria or mycobacterium.[2] The most important is the spectrum smear examination but false negative results are obtained because of :

1. Improper sputum specimen collection.
2. Defective slide preparation.
3. Washing off the material.
4. Faulty sputum fixation.
5. Under or over staining.
6. Improper slide examination.
7. Incompetent slide study.

Causative Agent

Mycobacterium tuberculosis is an aerobic organism, growing best at 7.4 pH and PO_2 of 100-140 mm of Hg; dividing almost every 16-20 hours. There may be 100 millions or more bacilli present in a cavitational lesion, and for any single mycobacterium tuberculosis, these may be 1:10000 or more single drug resistant mutants in addition to many more secondary resistant mutants, in those who have been inadequately treated.[2] Pulmonary tuberculosis generally presenting four types of patients:

1. Lesion exists extracellularly in cavities containing very actively and rapidly multiplying organisms, which become major sources of drug resistant organisms.
2. Extracellular closed caseous lesions, containing slowly or intermittently dividing organisms, giving rise to a population of persisters, hence justifying for prolonged therapy.
3. Intracellular within macrophages closed caseous lesion, containing few number of organisms, dividing occasionally.
4. Lesions with dormant bacilli which line as such for years and divide only when the immune system get weakened.

Curative Agents (Chemotherapy)

Conventional treatment lasting for one and a half years to two years has not proved beneficial, because of longer time involved, patient's noncompliance and lack of proper supervision for such a long period as well as irregularities by the patient regarding the drug and its dosages.[2] Short courses for treating

Table 15.1(a)[2,5]: Daily regimens

Recommended standard 6-month regimen
2 HRZ/4HR
Variants
2E (ORS) HRZ/4HR
3E (ORS) HRZ/3HR
6E (ORS HRZ
2SHRZ/6HT
3E (ORS) HRZ/6EHR
3E (ORS) HRZ/9EH

Table 15.1(b)[2,5]: Intermittent regimens

Regimen
3E (ORS) HRZ/6H_3R_3
3E (ORS) HRZ/6H_2R_2
3E (ORS) HRZ/9E_2H_2
3E (ORS_3) $H_3R_3Z_3$/6$E_3H_3R_3$
2HRZ/4H_3R_3
2HRZ/4H_2R_2
2$E_3H_3R_3Z_3$/4H_3R_3
2$S_3H_3R_3Z_3$/4H_3R_3
2SHRZ/6$S_2H_2Z_2$

S = Streptomycin H = Isoniazid R = Rifampicin
Z = Pyrazinamide E = Ethambutol T = Thiacetazone

Prefixed digit means number of months
Post fixed digit means number of days in a week

pulmonary tuberculosis usually lasting in months and mostly less than a year have proved to be successful[2,5] because of shorter period, easy availability of potent drugs, with an aim of nearly 100% results, therefore, better patient compliance. It is always started with 3-4 drugs at the initial intensive phase (continuation phase) with two to three drugs during the maintenance phase. Irrespective of daily regimen or intermittent regimen, triple drug therapy is suggested in the continuation phase, on the presumption that the patients are resistant to one or more drugs.[6] Short course treatment is not recommended if there are toxic reactions to isoniazid or rifampicin or both the drugs are found to be resistant.[2] Both daily and intermittent regimens are shown in the Tables 15.1a and 15.1b. There is no cross resistance between these commonly used drugs; only it exists between kanamycin and capreomycin and between ethionamide and thiacetazone.[5] Dosage schedule is shown in Table 15.2. Recommended drug dosage remain appropriate and applicable to all types of tuberculosis including miliary and meningitis and both for adults and children.[2,5]

Management of T in HN disease is essentially the same and once patient starts tolerating anti TB chemotherapy, anti retroviral therapy can be started alongwith. CD_4 cell count of more than 200 cells/cumm is usually considered safe. If CD_4 cells count is going below 50 cells/cumm, HAART should immediately be started. Adverse drug reactions should be look for, as these are more in TB with HIV disease and mostly in first month of initiation of treatment and in case these occur, offending drug needs to be immediately stopped.[7,8]

Management of Multi Drug Resistant (MDR-TB) requires aggressive approach with five or even six drugs and patient should be strictly followed. Never add single drug to the pre-existing regimen in case of failure. Surgical adjuvant therapy can help in few patients.

Table 15.2: Dosage schedule

Drug	Daily			Intermittent		
	Dosage Mg/Kg*	*Adult weight (kg)*	*Dose (mg)*	*Dosage (mg/kg)*	*Adults weight (kg)*	*Dose (mg)*
Isoniazid	5-8	—	300	15	—	850
Rifampicin	10-12	< 50 50	450 600	15	—	600 900
Pyrazinamide	35	<50 50	1500 2000	50 (Thrice a week) 75 (twice a week)	< 50 50 <50 50	2000 2500 3000 3500
Streptomycin	15-20 15-20	<50 50	750 1000	15-20 15-20	<50 50	750 1000
Ethambutol	25 × 2 month then 15	—	—	30 (thrice a week) 45 (thrice a week)	—	–

*1. Accurate dose calculations help ensure efficacy and avoid toxicity.
2. Dose for adults and children is same.

Interactions and Contraindications

Isoniazid interacts with phenytoin, carbamazepine and ethosuxamide. Rifampicin induces hepatic microsomal enzymes and reduces half life and clinical efficacy of oral hypoglycaemic agents, corticosteroids, digoxin, oral contraceptives, coumarin anticoagulants and dapsone when given concurrently.[2,5]

Pyrazinamide is contraindicated in gout, because it's metabolite pyrazinoic acid inhibits renal tubular secretion of uric acid, leading to hyperuricemia.[9]

Streptomycin is nephrotoxic in case of impaired renal functions. Because of its ototoxicity, better avoid in young babies, elderly patients, pregnant mothers and patients with myasthenia. Secondary risk (because of improper sterilisation of injecting needles) of transmitting viral diseases and AIDS does exist.[5] And ethambutol should be avoided in young children and in high risk patients, because of ocular toxicity.

Generalized Reactions[2]

A wide range is included in its clinical manifestation, where most common being rash and fever. Other signs and symptoms being conjunctivitis, periorbital oedema, nausea, vomiting, generalized aches, hepatosplenomegaly, lymphadenopathy, albuminuria, mild jaundice and rarely exfoliative dermatitis. For minor reactions, simple antihistaminic and reassurance will do, without stopping the chemotherapy. For a serious reaction, management includes identifying the drug responsible and remove; while adequate therapy with minimum of two drugs should be kept continued. Desensitization is necessary only when the drug responsible is essential for the regimen. Challenge does chart has been shown in Table 15.3. Hepatitis[8,9] is another generalized reaction to almost all the antitubercular drugs. But all hepatitis during antitubercular treatment may not be caused by the regimen, since chronic liver disease and infectious hepatitis are quite common in this part of the tropics; as coexisting entity. Mild, symptom free, transitory alteration (rise) in serum hepatic enzymes is a usual feature in early part of treatments but persistent symptoms of clinical hepatitis like vomiting, nausea, anorexia, jaundice and hepatomegaly require immediate stopping of the drug and institution of supportive treatment, although treatment with same drug regimen can be kept continued with proper monitoring liver function tests.

Table 15.3: *Challenge doses for detecting cutaneous or generalized hypersensitivity to antitubercular drugs

Drug	*Challenge dose*	
	Day 1	*Day 2*
Isoniazid	50 mg	300 mg
Rifampicin	75 mg	300 mg
Pyrazinamide	250 mg	1 gm
Ethambutol	100 mg	500 mg
Streptomycin or other aminoglycosides	125 mg	500 mg

* Reproduced from Bull. IUAT; 1984 59: 152-62 by Girling D.J. only for the commonly used drugs.

Adverse Effects[1,2,5]

Isoniazid—Cutaneous hypersensitivity, peripheral neuropathy, hepatitis.

Rarely—Giddiness, convulsion, haemolytic anaemia, aplastic anaemia, agranulocytosis, arthralgia, gynaecomastia.

Rifampicin—Cutaneous reactions, Gastrointestinal reactions, Hepatitis.

During Intermittent Therapy

a. Cutaneous syndrome—Rash, itching, flushing.
b. Abdominal syndrome—Nausea, vomiting, colic, diarrhoea.
c. Flu syndrome—Fever, chills, headache, bone pains.
d. Respiratory syndrome—Shortness of breath, collapse.
e. Miscellaneous—Thrombocytopenia leucopenia, purpura, haemolytic anaemia, acute renal failure.

Ethambutol—Hyperuricaemia, retrobulbar neuritis.

Rarely—Hepatitis, cutaneous hypersensitivity and peripheral neuropathy.

Pyrazinamide

a. Nausea, vomiting, flushing.
b. Arthralgia, hepatitis, cutaneous hypersensitivity.
c. *Rare*—Photosensitization, sideroblastic anaemia.

Streptomycin

a. Cutaneous hypersensitivity, giddiness, numbness, tinnitus.

b. Vertigo, ataxia, ototoxicity.

Rarely: Renal toxicity, aplastic anaemia, agranulocytosis.

To patients with impaired renal functions these three drugs namely isoniazid, pyrazinamide and rifampicin can safely be given but not with impaired hepatic functions, where a close monitoring of liver functions is required.[9,10] All drugs can be given safely during pregnancy except for streptomycin and same is true for diabetic patients except for monitoring of blood glucose which requires more of the oral hypoglycaemic agents because of coadministration of rifampicin.[10,11]

REFERENCES

1. Bhatia R.S., Antitubercular drugs adverse reactions; Antiseptic 1987;84:142-45.
2. Aziz A. Update management of pulmonary tuberculosis; proceedings of XV eastern region conference of IUAT and LB: 1987;49-59.
3. WHO technical report series N. 290;1964; Geneva.
4. Fox W., Whither short course chemotherapy; Bull. IUAT; 1981;56:135-55.
5. Girling D.J. Anti TB regimens of chemotherapy—Recommendations from the committee on treatment of IUAT and LD; Proceedings of XV eastern region conference of IUAT and LD; 1987:65-72.
6. Aziz A., Ishaw M, Jaffar N.A., Akhwant R and Bhatti A.M., Clinical trial of two short course regimens and a standard regimen chemotherapy in retreatment of pulmonary tuberculosis in Pakistan; results 18 months after completion of treatment: Am. Rev. Resp. Dis., 1986;134:1056-61.
7. Bhatia R.S., HIV and TB: The ominous connection: In. PC Manoria ed. PG Med API, 1998;12:104-07.
8. Swaminanthan S., *et al.* Extrapulmonary TB; In: SB Gupta; ed. Med Update: API 2005;15:653-58.
9. Bhatia R.S, Comparative study of hepatic toxicity of two drug—regimens with and without pyrazinamide; Medicine and Surgery; 1987;27:13-14.
10. Bhatia R.S, Update management of pulmonary TB; The Ind; Practitioner 1991;527-32.
11. Bhatia R.S., Adverse reactions to rifampicin; IJCP; 1991;11:57-69.

Chapter sixteen

Management Strategies in Co-existing Tuberculosis and HIV Disease

RS Bhatia

ABSTRACT

The centuries old disease tuberculosis has emerged as the most common opportunistic infection in HIV infected patients. The dual infection adds morbidity, where HIV infection helps in spreading the tuberculosis and the interaction between the two has lethal implications. Tuberculosis in HIV disease brings forth many issues such as atypical presentations posing diagnostic difficulties, drug-drug interaction and paradoxical reactions posing treatment difficulties and emerging MDR-TB and occurrence of polymicrobial infections such as pneumocystis carinii pneumonia, cytomegalovirus and other bacterial infections posing management difficulties, especially in the advance disease. Tuberculosis assumes particular importance for its contagious spread by inhalation and readily treatability with present effective drugs that are required to be used effectively in full dose and for appropriate duration.

INTRODUCTION

Poor and (over)populated societies have high prevalence of tuberculosis, even upto 80% of adults carrying TB germ in overcrowded cities of some developing countries.[1] And 9% of total 8.3 million new TB adult cases are attributable to HIV infection, the risk of developing active TB is increased by 25-30 times than those with mycobacterium infection alone.[2] Again out of 1.8 million deaths this from TB, 12% are attributable to HIV, where TB remains the immediate cause of 11% of adult deaths in AIDS.[3] And out of 52,000 deaths due to TB every week, more than 40% occur in Southeast Asia. Tuberculosis is a major health problem in Southeast Asia[4] infecting 40-50% of nearly 6 million adults living with HIV disease in this region . Due to interaction of HIV and TB, prevalence of extra pulmonary TB may increase from 15% to 70% especially when CD cell count is decreased to 100 cells/mm^3.[4,5,6] Diagnostic difficulties of TB in HIV disease occur because of the following features such as extrapulmonary presentation, AFB negativity, Tuberculin test negativity or weak response and lower and middle zone involvement. There is an increased risk to community alongwith concomitant emergence of MDR-TB.[7]

Due to constraints of laboratory facilities in India, using tuberculin test positively with cut off criterion of 2 mm induration,[8] the sensitivity of the test can be significantly utilized in early detection of mycobacterial infection amongst HIV positive individuals, especially when CD_4 cell count is not possible.[9] The positive tuberculin test when stratified by induration measured reveals positivity of test (2 mm induration) in HIV +ve cases in 80% as compared to 24% in HIV -ve cases.[8]

CLINICAL PICTURE

Clinical features are most atypical, where lungs are less affected and the disease is more disseminated to other organs. Chest X-ray findings are given in Table 16.1. Sputum smear and stool smear are positive for AFB hardly in 40% of cases. This necessitates the need for more sensitive and rapid diagnostic tests. The dual infection has pulmonary involvement in 74-100% of cases and physical findings are indistinguishable between those with and those without HIV infection, posing a lost of difficulty in differential diagnosis. Extrapulmonary involvement in the form of lymphadenitis, miliary or disseminated tuberculosis, has been included as AIDS indicator of disease in the Indian context.[10] HIV disease with tuberculosis can present as chronic meningitis with headache and altered sensorium. Fever and signs of meningeal irritation are less common.

Table 16.1: Chest X-ray findings in pulmonary TB in association with HIV infection

Hilar lymphadenopathy	42%
Pleural effusion	29%
Upper lobe infiltrates	25%
Miliary pattern	13%
Cavitation	0.6%

Diagnosis

Diagnosis is difficult in AIDS since TB has unusual presentation and lacks simultaneous histologic reaction in some cases due to depressed cell mediated immunity. Tuberculin test is no longer recommended for routine use in TB screening programme of HIV infected persons. The results of anergy testing using a panel of antigens give inconsistent and ambiguous observations. The test positivity of 5 mm induration in HIV and TB co-infection with CD_4 count > 500 cells/mm^3 as 50-90% may fall to 0-20% with CD_4 cell count falling to < than 200 cells/mm^3. Those with relatively well preserved cell immunity (manifested by positive tuberculin test and lack of other HIV associated infections), chest findings are similar to those of reactivation TB in immunocompetent patients, including cavitation and upper lobe infiltration. In contrast, those with immunosuppression due to HIV infection have chest findings that are typical of primary TB in immunocompetent patients such as hilar lymphadenopathy, miliary TB and pleural effusion. Disease other than TB can give both classical and atypical findings on chest X-ray and in cases with sputum smear negativity, other differentials, especially the HIV related pulmonary diseases such as bacterial pneumonia, pneumocystic carinii pneumonia, kaposi's sarcoma, fungal infections and nocardiosis have to be considered. Sputum positivity for AFB may vary from 31-82%.[11] The positivity of AFB falls to 5% in HIV infected patients with pulmonary tuberculosis, although it forms cornerstone of diagnosis of TB even in high HIV prevalence areas. All types of pleural involvement may occur. Those with isolated unilateral involvement may have better prognosis.[12] Multi drug resistant TB (MDR-TB) is caused by a strain of mycobacterium tuberculosis that is resistant to two or more antitubercular drugs, usually isoniazid and rifampicin. It is a serious problem and case fatality in HIV with MDR-TB is 70% in 4-6 weeks as compared to non HIV with MDR-TB where it is 25%. MDR-TB associated with HIV infection is being labelled as the third epidemic that is one of the most malignant of opportunistic infections.

Primary resistance in developing countries like India is 15%. Acquired resistance from initial response is constantly increasing and this problem shall further worsen with HIV endemicity. In MDR-TB, risk factors include inadequate treatment; non-compliance, especially in lower socio-economic patients, presence of cavitary lesions, HIV infection, IV drug use, following anticancer therapy and after organ transplant.

Mechanism of development of resistance includes:

a. Natural resistance due to spontaneous mutation.
b. Primary resistance through infection with resistant tubercle bacilli.
c. Acquired resistance in those have inadequate therapy, this being the strongest predictor for MDR-TB.
d. Initially resistance may be seen in those who have taken the chemotherapy intentionally or unintentionally. Extra pulmonary diseases are upto 70% in HIV related TB if the CD cell count is < than 100/ mm^3. Diagnosis of extra pulmonary TB is often difficult. Variety of diagnostic tests have to be indicated depending on the site of infection.

Pathogenesis

In an immunocompetent person on infection with *M. tuberculosis*, the organism is presented in the macrophage through ingestion, thereafter the processed mycobacterial antigens are presented to T-cells. The CD_4 cells secrete lymphokines that enhance the capacity of macrophage to ingest and kill the mycobacteria. In majority of the people, the infection is contained and TB does not develop, although a number of dormant bacilli remain in the body. Only 10% of cases develop clinical TB, soon after primary infection or years later as reactivation TB. The consequences in the HIV positive background are possibly due to defects in T cells and/or macrophages functions.[11]

Progressive depletion and dysfunction of CD_4 cells, coupled with defects in macrophage and monocyte function, form the hallmark of HIV infection. An epidemiological evidence favours that HIV infection increases the risk of reactivation of latent TB and also the risks of progressive disease from new infection.[13,14]

Treatment

Treatment of TB aims at curing the patient alongwith minimizing the transmission of mycobacterium tuberculosis to the community. The recommendations for the treatment remain the same for TB in HIV infected or uninfected patients.

Intermittent regimens are contraindicated, adherence strategies including DOT are given importance and drug-drug interaction is strictly observed for better compliance and results. Hepatotoxicity is always looked for being a serious obstacle. Effective treatment with four drugs (rifampicin, isoniazid, ethambutol and pyrazinamide) for two months, followed by three drugs for seven months without pyazinamide, gives 80% conversion after three months of treatment. However, relapses have been reported, but mortality, if occurs, is due to other opportunistic infections. Adverse reactions to drugs are more frequent in these cases; 90% of these occur in the first two months. In treating MDR-TB, a five drug regimen has been suggested, while treating MDR-TB in HIV patients, even six drugs have been suggested to be used. There is a need to add two new drugs instead of one.

A case control study in a large New York City Hospital that included MDR-TB cases with and without HIV revealed that five or six drugs combination that was used included either of the following additional drugs:

1. Capreomycin plus ciprofloxacin.
2. Capreomycin plus cycloserine.
3. Ciprofloxacin + cycloserine + capreomycin.

In meningeal tuberculosis in HIV disease, in areas where initial resistance is less than 4%, three to four drugs combination for a minimum of 12 months is necessary but 50% of patients may need longer treatment which is essential because of concurrent HIV disease. In case of infection with MDR-TB, more than five drugs including ciprofloxacin, clofazimine, clarithromycin or cyclosporine should be dispensed. It has to be differentiated from *M. avium* complex infection, typically presenting as mass lesions such as tuberculoma, cerebral or spinal cord abscess. Prevention of these infections, both TB and AIDS—the ancient and modern plagues which dare to raise their ugly heads, can only be done through public awareness and education regarding correct behavior and code of conduct in human sexual needs. While treating the patients with HIV disease, the aim is maximal suppression of HIV replication for as long as possible. Three-drug combination of two nucleoside analogues with a protease inhibitor (PI), initiated early in the course of HIV infection forms the current standard care of HIV patients.[15] In India, 2 NRI and one NNRI combination is the choice drug. If CD_4 cell count is below 50/mm^3, HAART has to be started, if less than 200/mm^3, HAART should be started and if more than 200 mm^3, it is better to complete anti Koch's treatment or initial intensive therapy at least. HAART is started only as soon as anti TB therapy is tolerated.[16] Patients with CD_4 cells count more than 200/mm^3 have a low risk. ZDV/dd1/3TC combination triple therapy is less potent, more complicating hepatotoxicity. ZDV (or dMT) 3TC/EF2 is another option for patients being coadministered rifampicin. Another option for PI containing combinations of ZDV/3TC/SQV/r or d4T/3TC/SQV/r with concomitant use of rifampicin is in offing where dose of ritonavir should be 400 mg twice a day.

Drug interaction is less pronounced with some protease inhibitors with refabutin but it is available only in resource limited setting. Paradoxical reaction/ immune reconstitution of inflammatory syndrome (IRIS) appears to occur more commonly initiation of HAART and not because of anti TB treatment, generally within 15 days (median) and mostly in patients with advanced HIV infection[17] where CD_4 cell count is less than 50/mm^3. This happens in 36% of patients receiving antiretroviral therapy along with anti TB drugs as compared to 7% in patients receiving anti TB drugs alone, in the form of worsening of pleuro pulmonary lesions, cutaneous and psoas abscess, effusions in pleura, peritoneum and pericardium, tuberculoma and lymphadenopathy. Life threatening IRIS such as meningitis, raised intracranial tension and pulmonary opacities leading to ARDS require urgent corticosteroids.

Chemoprophylaxis

Public education regarding correct sexual behaviour forms the cornerstone, in preventing this dual infection. Chemoprophylaxis of healthy contacts is highly important. Chemoprophylaxis with isoniazid alone may not look to be a prudent step. Five mm induration instead of 10 mm should be the criterion for positive tuberculin test. So, criteria for isoniazid chemoprophylaxis has been suggested to be either tuberculin test of more than five mm induration with 5 IU or CD_4 cell count below 200/cu mm, and prophylaxis is recommended for 12 months for any person of any age. Nosocomial infection of tuberculosis to indoor patients and to health care workers adds gravity to hospitalized morbidity and burden on health care agencies respectively. These infections especially MDR-TB have been recorded even as an outbreak by CDC in health departments of Florida and New York city. That is why CDC and American Thoracic Society have recommended preventive therapy especially in patients exposed to MDR-TB to decrease the risk of active disease. This includes use of ciprofloxacin

750 mg BD or ofloxacin 400 mg or pyrazinamide 35 mg/kg/day for contacts deemed likely to be newly infected with MDR-TB and at high risk for active disease.

BCG is beneficial in HIV infection in preventing the TB infection and putting aside the theoretical fear of disseminating TB infection in HIV infected infants. BCG vaccination should be given to all infants even when the mother is a known suspected case of HIV infection; however, BCG should be withheld from patients with symptomatic HIV infection.

AIDS vaccine trials and their evaluation have been entrusted to NARI of ICMR. There are certain difficulties such as maintenance of high level immune response and variability of virus. Ideal HIV vaccine would be that, which works against all the major five subtypes of the virus.[18,19] Trials have been started recently. We have to wait for their results.

Comments

Deficient cell mediated immunity is the common denominator, both for tuberculosis and HIV disease. More than 50% of AIDS cases suffer from tuberculosis in India. HIV infection and tuberculosis relationship is exhibited in Table 16.2. Reactivation of tuberculosis is common in early HIV disease. Clinical presentation and response to anti-tubercular therapy is similar to non HIV-tubercular disease. Progressive HIV disease with severe immuno-deficiency leads to extrapulmonary and disseminated tuberculosis requiring aggressive and prolonged treatment. Incidence of multi-drug resistant tuberculosis has increased. MAC infection is often a late opportunistic infection. Six or even more drugs combination including fluoroquines is recommended for combating MDR-tuberculosis.[20] Although, sparfloxacin has shown dose related activity both in vivo and in vitro,[21] a caution has been given to use it in MDR-TB[22] only after extended human studies are undertaken. Prevention of MDR-TB is more important than treating the same.[23,24]

Table 16.2: TB and HIV infection

1. Reactivation common
2. Difficult diagnosis
3. Poor prognosis
4. Extra pulmonary lesions of TB
5. MDR—TB

REFERENCES

1. UNAIDS: TB and AIDS, UNAIDS point of view, UNAIDS best practice collections; Oct. 1997.
2. How do TB and HIV infect in individuals; AIDS Update 1996;2(2)):1.
3. Corbett EL *et al.*; The growing burden of TB: Global trends and interaction with the HIV epidemics; Arch. Intern Med: 2003;163:1009-21.

4. Patel AK, Patel KK; HIV and TB; In: SB Gupta; ed: Med. Update, API, 2005;15:726-30.
5. Balasubramanian R, Ramachandran R; Management of non pulmonary forms of TB; Ind. J Paed 2000;67:34-40.
6. Swaminathan S, Narendran G; Extrapulmonary TB; In: SB Gupta, ed; Med. Update API 2005;15:653-58.
7. WHO: Guidelines for implementing Collaborative TB and HIV programme activities; WHO report, Geneva WHO 2003.
8. Velhal GB, Bichile SK. Tuberculin test in HIV positive individual. JAPI 1998;46:989-90.
9. Girija Singh, Pais. Tuberculin sensitivity in HIV seropositives with TB compared to seronegatives. JAPI 1998;46:1029-30.
10. Banarjee K. HIV/AIDS—Criteria of diagnosis. An overview: In: YP Munjal; ed. Medicine Update API 1997;7:497-503.
11. Mahashur AA; TB and HIV infection. In: PS Shankar ed Pulm Tuber: A JAPI production. The National Book Depot, Parel, Mumbai 1995;36-39.
12. Gupta KB, *et al*. Pleural involvement in patients coinfected with HIV and M. tuberculosis: Clinico radiological profile: Lung India 1999;17(2):65-67.
13. Bhatia RS, Bedi PS, Sibia SS, HIV infection and TB. TB Update 1997; 1:14-16.
14. Johnson JL, et al. Duration of efficiency of treatment of latent TB infection in HIV-infected adults; AIDS 2001:15:2137-47.
15. Vajpayee M, Dar L. Anti retroviral drugs in HIV infection. Ind J Pharm 1999;31(2):96-103.
16. Dean GL *et al*: Treatment of TB in HIV infected persons in the era of highly active anti-retroviral therapy; AIDS 2002;16:75-83.
17. Pozniak A; BHIVA treatment guidelines for TB/HIV infection; HIV Med; 2003;Suppl 1:1-41.
18. Jayasingh RS. Vaccine update In: YP Munjal; ed; Med Update: API 1997;7:856-62.
19. Bhatia RS. HIV and TB: The ominous connection, In: PC Manoria, ed: PG Med API, Mumbai 1998;12(III):104-107.
20. Alanzaden Gj, Lerner SA. The clinical use of fluoroquinolones for the treatment of mycobacterial diseases. Clin Inf Dis 1997:25:1213-21.
21. Shankar PS. Sparfloxacin in tuberculosis: Editorial JAPI; 1998:46:759-60.
22. Bhatia RS, Sibia SS. Treatment of tuberculosis: Role of sparfloxacin? JAPI 1999;47:750.
23. National consensus on MDR-TB tuberculosis: Research forum. Lung India 1999;17(2):57-64.
24. Bhatia RS; Tuberculosis and acquired immunodeficiency syndrome: JAPI:2000;48:613-16.

Chapter seventeen

Current Aspects in the Surgical Management of Tuberculosis

SK Sarkar

INTRODUCTION

With the progressive discovery of antimicrobial drugs the role of surgery in the treatment of Pulmonary Tuberculosis has declined.[1-5] In India, there are however 2 million new cases of active tuberculosis being reported annually, among these there remain about 2% of patients who require surgical consideration.

Currently there is a significant increase in the incidence of drug-resistant organisms, including both Mycobacterium tuberculosis and atypical strains, and this accounts for the majority of surgical cases today. The role of surgery also lies in the management of pulmonary complications like severe hemoptysis, chronic emphysema, bronchiectasis, scar carcinoma etc.

Principles of Surgical Procedures

Surgical treatment of pulmonary tuberculosis is based on mainly 3 principles:

1. Collapse therapy (Artificial pneumothorax, pneumoperitoneum, thoracoplasty).
2. Excisional surgery (Pulmonary resections).
3. Drainage procedures (Cavernostomy, Monaldi).

Collapse Therapy

This can be compared to a splint or a crutch for protection of an injured extremity. The objectives of this therapy include:

i. Restriction of lung movements.
ii. Reduction of lung cavities.
iii. Closure of lung cavities.
iv. Reduction of thoracic space volume especially in post-resectional cases.

Collapse therapy may be of temporary or permanent type. Temporary methods include artificial pneumothorax, pneumoperitoneum and phrenic nerve crushing for paralyzing diaphragm. The procedure of artificial pneumothorax received widespread popularity after reporting of a successful case series by Forlanini (1882 and 1894) and John B. Murphy (1898). This method is now being used sporadically in patients with pulmonary tuberculosis. Pneumoperitoneum was introduced by Banyal (1931) and popularized by Vadja (1933). There is no permanent loss of lung function and the procedure is still of choice for the purpose of relaxing a diseased lower table.

Thoracoplasty

It is a permanent method to relax or compress the tuberculous lung. Eastlander first used the term “Thoracoplasty” in 1879 to denote removal of ribs so as to collapse the chest wall down to the lung, which would not expand after drainage of an empyema. In 1885, Decerenvilli first used this operation to collapse the cavity in a tuberculous lung. Brauers (1907) suggested sub periosteal resection of the ribs, and multistage operation to reduce the paradox of the flail portion of the chest wall and it further was modified by Sauerbruch, Gourdet and Wilms.

Alexander (1937)[6] refined the “Modern” operation of thoracoplasty and reported 11 percent mortality, with cavity closure in 93% of the survivors.

Indications, Contraindications and Thoracoplasty

The majority of the patients requiring surgical care are successfully treated by resection, but thoracoplasty is still justified in certain “Salvage Cases”, in which resection is not possible because of bilateral extensive disease with highly productive drug resistant organisms and poor cardio respiratory reserve.[7,8] Thoracoplasty is done in chemotherapy failure drug resistant cases, cases with persistently positive sputum for acid fast bacilli with hemoptysis, cavities in the lung apex which are “not” too medial, too big, too thin or under tension.

The use of combined thoracoplasty with intercostals myoplasty for treating chronic empyema has been reported by Hellar[9] and Wangenstein[10] and were modified by grow.[11] This method is still of choice in treating chronic empyema with or without bronchopleural fistula where resectional surgery is not possible. The results were rewarding and there was no mortality as reported in an earlier study of 171 patients by us.[12]

Resection (Excision) Therapy

This method is the nearest approach to curative treatment of pulmonary tuberculosis in association with adequate chemotherapy. Freelander performed the first successful complete lobectomy for tuberculosis in 1934. In 1953, Chamberlain[13] and associates presented a series of 300 segmental resections for pulmonary tuberculosis with an operative mortality of 3 percent.

Indications for Resection

The purpose of surgery is to remove, or to assist in the healing, or the control of destructive residuals that would otherwise contribute to the failure of medical treatment or to the reactivation of the disease process. The indications include:

1. Residual caseous necrotic foci should be removed because of the fear of subsequent spread of disease when the focus becomes liquefied and establishes bronchial communication.
2. An open cavity with positive sputum beyond six months of continuous chemotherapy.
3. Persistent positive sputum cultures after six months of chemotherapy in patients without demonstrable cavitation but with pathological results, such as a destroyed lobe or lung, localized bronchiectasis, bronchial stenosis with resultant atelectasis.
4. Patients with negative sputum who have a residual destroyed segment, lobe of lung and blocked cavities. There is threat of reactivation of tuberculosis and troublesome hemoptysis in such cases if not treated surgically.
5. The presence of localized infection with atypical group III (Battey) organisms is an acceptable indication for resection because of the organisms' primary resistance to drugs.
6. Tubercular bronchiectasis of the middle and lower lobes have got a poor drainage and are advised to be resected.
7. Suspected presence of a concomitant neoplasm within a tuberculous lesion.
8. Recurrent or persistent life threatening hemoptysis may require emergency resection.
9. Patients with pleural empyema with spontaneous bronchopleural fistula or any postoperative bronchopleural, fistula may need resection as well as a decortication.
10. Tuberculoma of lung.
11. MDR tuberculosis.

Contraindications for Resection

Indications for operation in pulmonary tuberculosis must be tempered by various specific contraindications, such as inadequate cardio-pulmonary reserve, ventilatory insufficiency, presence of another debilitating disease with poor prognosis, generalized or extra pulmonary tuberculosis that is progressive despite adequate chemotherapy and presence of active arteriosclerotic heart disease. Active endobronchial tuberculosis and associated lung carcinoma, that cannot be controlled by operation may obviate operative intervention.

Selection of Patients and Pre-operative Management

Thoracoplasty should not be planned in growing children and young adults. Younger patients tolerate resection better. Young women and adolescent girls are prone to recurrence of arrested tuberculosis and hence they may need "Curative" resectional surgery. Resection may be recommended in patients with thick walled cavities, patients who have responded slowly, as determined by sputum conversion and by lack of radiographic improvement, patients who are likely to be unreliable in taking medicine or obtaining follow up examination, such as alcoholics and drug addicts. Occupation and the economic status of the patient particularly in men play an important role. Patients, with poor socioeconomic and poor educational resource must perform strenuous labour for their livelihood requires a more definitive treatment.

An effort should be made to convert the patient's sputum to negative as far as possible (with 6 to 8 months of continuous possible emergence of drug resistance. Preoperative evaluation for all patients undergoing surgical treatment should include measures to improve branchial hygiene through the use of bronchodilators, nebulised mists and appropriate antibiotic therapy.

Pulmonary function studies with determination of arterial blood gas levels are helpful, particularly in the borderline cases. In selected cases bronchograms and CT scans are useful in demonstrating unsuspected bronchiectasis and in delineating the diseased segments. Fibreoptic bronchoscopy should be performed in all patients to demonstrate the unsuspected presence of endobronchial tuberculosis, bronchostenosis or other nontuberculous endobronchial lesions.

Improvement of nutritional status and anemia can be achieved by adding high protein, high caloric diet along with vitamin C and iron preparations.

Complications of Surgery and Management

The complications can be avoided or minimized by correct timing of the operative procedure, meticulous surgical technique and rapid re-expansion of remaining lung tissue. The usual complications of thoracotomy can be avoided by meticulous postoperative care, use of proper antibiotics and maintenance of fluid balance. The most distressing postoperative complications appearing with some frequency in tubercular patients include bronchopleural fistula and empyema.

Bronchopleural Fistula

In about 3 to 7% patients of pulmonary tuberculosis undergone resectional surgery, bronchopleural fistula has been reported in the literature.[14,15] This complication usually occurs at the end of first week after surgery. Patients may complain of fever and blood tinged sputum. Skiagram shows presence of air or air fluid level in the pleural cavity or there may be continuous air leak via the intercostal catheter for more than two weeks. Tension pneumothorax may develop in some cases. This complication may occur as a result of poor surgical technique in closing the stump, infection of the stump by tubercular micobacteria or non-tubercular organism, or sometimes due to poor healing as in old age, marked debility and after radiation therapy.

The cardinal rule in the management of broncho-pleural fistula is the establishment of pleural drainage. If fistula becomes apparent within three to four days of the initial resection an immediate operative reclosure is justified. Unfortunately, most fistulas do not become apparent until several weeks following resection and in such cases consideration is given to the appropriate timing of a tailoring thoracoplasty to obliterate the pleural space. If this is not successful in closing the fistula, a myoplasty utilizing a flap based on the intercostal muscles[10-12] or pectoral muscles[16,17] may be employed with excellent result.

CONCLUSIONS

Pulmonary tuberculosis still remains a global threat. An increasing number of patients with multi-drug resistant tuberculosis require resectional surgery along with second line anti-tuberculosis chemotherapy in the 21st century.[18,19] The clinical judgment of the treating surgeon remains the final decision. In our opening the continuing role of thoracoplasty still exists in treating localized cavitary disease with persistent positive sputum.

REFERENCES

1. Harrison LH. Current aspects of the surgical management of Tuberculosis. Surg Clin North Am 1980;60:883-95.
2. Weissbery D, Refacly Y. The place of surgery in the treatment of re-emerging pulmonary tuberculosis. Ann Ital Chir 2001;71:649-52.
3. Neptune WB, Kin S, Bookwalter J. Current surgical management of pulmonary tuberculosis. J. Thorac. and Cardiovasc. Surg. 1970;60:384-91.
4. Mc Laughlin JS, Hankin JR. Current aspects of surgery for pulmonary tuberculosis, Ann. Thorac. Surg. 1974;27:513-25.
5. Byrd RB, Kaplau PO, Gracey DR. Treatment of pulmonary tuberculosis. Chest 1974;66:560-67.
6. Alexander J. The surgery of pulmonary tuberculosis. Philadelphia and New York, Lea and Febiger, 1925.
7. Sabiston DC Jr, Spencer FC. Gibbons surgery of the chest, Fourth edition. W.B. Saunders and Company, Philadelphia 1983;1(20):612.
8. Sarkar SK, Bhatnagar M, Mathur A, Yadav KS, Sharma TN. Continuing role of thoracoplasty for pulmonary tuberculosis: Review of 155 cases. Ind J Thor Cradiovasc Surg 1989-90;6:62-65.
9. Heller E, Ueber Verhutung and Behandlung der Empyema Restholen. Chirug, 1934;6:3.
10. Wangenstein OH. The pedicled muscle flap in the closure of persistent bronchopleural fistula. J. Thorac. Surg 1935;5:27-53.
11. Grow JB. Chronic pleural empyema Dis. Chest 1946;12:26.

12. Sarkar SK, Sharma TN, Singh H, Singh A, Purohit SD, Sharma VK. Thoracoplasty with intercostal myoplasty for closure of an empyema cavity and bronchopleural fistula. International Surgery 1985;70:219-21.
13. Chamberlain JM, Storey CF, Klopstock R, Daniels CF. Segmental resection for pulmonary tuberculosis (300 cases). J. Thorac. Surg. 1953;26:471.
14. Das PB, David JG. Excisional surgery in the treatment of pulmonary tuberculosis. 1977;69:217.
15. Hankins JR, Miller JE, Attar S. *et al*. Bronchopleural fistula: J. Thorac, Cardiovasc. Surg 1978;76:755.
16. Hankins JR, Miller JE, McLaughlin JS. The use of chest wall muscle flaps to close bronchopleural fistula: Experience with 21 patients, Ann. Thorac, Surg. 1978:25:491.
17. Pairolero PC, Arnold PG, Piehler JM. Intrathoracic transposition of extra thoracic skeletal muscle. J. Thorac. Cardiovasc. Surg 1983;86:809-17.
18. Shiraishi Y, Nakajema Y, Katsuragi N, Kurai M, Takashasti M. Resectional Surgery Combined with Chemotherapy remains the treatment of choice for multidrug-resistant tuberculosis. J Thorac Cardiovasc Surg 2004;128:523-28.
19. Chan ED, Laurel V, Strand MJ, Chan JF, Huynh MN, Goble M, *et al*. Treatment and outcome analysis of 205 patients with multidrug-resistant tuberculosis. Am J Respir Crit Care Med 2004;169:1103.

Chapter eighteen

Management of TB in Special Situations

NK Jain, Vijay Agarwal

Tuberculosis is a common problem worldwide. There is an alarming increase in the number of tuberculosis patients with the advent of HIV infection, especially in developing countries. Tuberculosis management is never a simple endeavor; it requires additional considerations in the following special situations. HIV, liver disease, pediatric TB, pregnancy, renal failure etc.

Chronic Renal Failure

Patients with chronic renal failure undergoing hemodialysis are at 10- to 25-fold increased risk of developing active tuberculosis (TB) once infected, compared to the general population. Unfortunately, these patients are also at increased risk of development of drug resistance due to the difficulty in managing their tuberculosis disease. These patients require careful monitoring for treatment of tuberculosis, drug-resistant tuberculosis in particular. Data regarding clearance of anti-tuberculosis drugs are best documented for patients with Creatinine clearance less than 30 ml/minute or for those undergoing hemodialysis. For individuals with mild renal failure or undergoing peritoneal dialysis, the data are less clear. In addition to the effects on drug clearance, the diseases that cause renal failure and concomitant treatments can also impact drug levels (by altering absorption or drug interactions). Table 18.1 describes dosing changes for patients with renal insufficiency.

Table 18.1: Dosing recommendations for adult patients with reduced renal function
and for adult patients receiving hemodialysis

Drug	*Change in frequency*	*Recommended doses and frequency for patients with creatinine clearance of < 30 ml/min or patient receiving hemodialysis*
Isoniazid	No change	300 mg once daily, or 900 mg 3 times/week
Rifampin	No change	600 mg once daily, or 600 mg 3 times/week
Pyrazinamide	Yes	25-35 mg/kg/dose 3 times/week (not daily)
Ethambutol	Yes	15-25 mg/kg/dose 3 times/week (not daily)

Contd.

Contd.

Levofloxacin	Yes	750-1000 mg/dose 3 times/week (not daily)
Cycloserine	Yes	250 mg once daily, or 500 mg/dose 3 times/week*
Ethionamide	No change	250-500 mg/dose daily
PAS	No change	4 gm/dose twice daily
Streptomycin	Yes	12-15 mg/kg/dose 2-3 times/week (not daily)
Capreomycin	Yes	12-15 mg/kg/dose 2-3 times/week (not daily)
Kanamycin	Yes	12-15 mg/kg/dose 2-3 times/week (not daily)
Amikacin	Yes	12-15 mg/kg/dose 2-3 times/week (not daily)

- Standard doses are given unless there is intolerance.
- The medications should be given after hemodialysis on the day of hemodialysis.
- Monitoring of serum drug concentrations should be considered to ensure adequate drug absorption, without excessive accumulation, and to assist in avoiding toxicity.
- There should be careful monitoring for evidence of neurotoxicity.
- Data currently are not available for patients receiving peritoneal dialysis. Until data become available, begin with doses recommended for patients receiving hemodialysis and verify adequacy of dosing using serum concentration monitoring.
- Dose the aminoglycosides, pyrazinamide, and ethambutol by Ideal Body Weight for obese patients.

Ideal Body Weight (Men): 50 kg plus 2.3 kg/inch over 5 feet.
Ideal Body Weight (Women): 45 kg plus 2.3 kg/inch over 5 feet.

Estimated Creatinine clearance calculations
Men: Ideal Body Weight (kg) × (140–age)/72 × serum creatinine (mg/dl).
Women: 0.85 × Ideal Body Weight (kg) × (140 – age)/72 × serum creatinine (mg/dl).

Liver Disease

All the antituberculosis drugs, with the exception of streptomycin[1] and possibly ethambutol, cycloserine and capreomycin[2,3] can cause, or have been associated with an elevation in the liver enzymes. In addition, many tuberculosis patients have evidence of underlying liver disease of various causes, the most frequent being alcohol related. In some patients frank hepatitis may result from treatment.

Elevation of serum transaminase in asymptomatic patients taking isoniazid,[4,5] Rifampicin[6] and also ethionamide[7] may be self limiting which poses the problem of whether these drugs should be stopped in patients showing such abnormalities. Risk factors for antituberculosis drugs-induced hepatotoxicity include increasing age, indiscriminate use of drugs, alcohol intake, acute or chronic liver disease, female sex, malnutrition and more advanced tuberculosis.

To define drugs-induced hepatotoxicity following criteria can be used:

a. A rise to five or greater than five times the normal level of ALT and/or AST ($\geq$ 200 U/L).
b. A rise in the level of serum total Bilirubin over 1.5 mg/dl.
c. Any increase in AST and/or ALT above pretreatment level together with anorexia, nausea, vomiting and jaundice.
d. Normalization of liver enzymes level and resolution of signs and symptoms of hepatotoxicity after withdrawal of all hepatotoxic drugs.

The Joint Tuberculosis Committee of British Thoracic Society recommended following guidelines[8] for the management of drugs-induced hepatotoxicity:

1. All tuberculosis patients should have pretreatment measurement of liver function.
2. Standard drug treatment should be given under the supervision of a respiratory or other suitably qualified physician.
3. All patients should be informed of possible side effects.
4. Regular monitoring of liver function is required in patients with known chronic liver disease e.g. alcoholic liver disease, chronic active hepatitis, cirrhosis and hepatitis B or C antigen positive.
5. If the patient has no evidence of pre-existing liver disease and normal pre-treatment liver function, liver function need only be repeated (and treatment stopped). If fever, malaise, vomiting, jaundice or unexplained deterioration during treatment occurs.
6. If the AST or ALT levels are two or more times above normal, liver function should be monitored weekly for two weeks and then two weekly until normal. If the AST or ALT levels are just under twice the normal values, liver function should be monitored two weekly.
7. If the patient is not unwell, and the form of tuberculosis is non-infectious, no treatment to be given until liver functions return to normal.
   If the patient is clinically unwell or the sputum is smear positive within two weeks of commencing treatment, then some drug therapy need to be given, preferably as an inpatient, until liver function is normal. Streptomycin, ethambutol and reserve drugs (like quinolones, macrolides) should be used.
   Once liver function is normal challenge dose of the original drugs can be reintroduced sequentially in the order isoniazid. Rifampicin and pyrazinamide with daily monitoring of patients clinical condition and liver function test. However, looking to high incidence of hepatic toxicity with Rifampicin in Indian sub-continent compared to low incidence of hepatic toxicity with Pyrazinamide and isoniazid,[9] sequence of reintroduction of these drugs should be isoniazid, Pyrazinamide and Rifampicin.
8. If there is no further reaction standard chemotherapy can be continued and any alternative drugs introduced temporarily can be withdrawn.

9. If there is a further reaction, the offending drug should be excluded and a suitable alternative regimen should be used.
10. Occasionally the choice of alternative drugs is so limited that desensitization and reintroduction of the offending drug may be necessary using conventional protocols.

Pregnancy

TB treatment should not be suspended because of pregnancy or lactation. The initial standard regimens may be administered with certain precautions. Streptomycin may cause ototoxicity to the fetus and, therefore, must be avoided.[8-10] The use of pyrazinamide during pregnancy is accepted worldwide but has not been approved by the FDA. Fluoroquinolones have been reported to interfere with fetal cartilage development and, therefore, must not be used during pregnancy. No teratogenic effects are associated with INH and rifampin.[8,11] Ethionamide is teratogenic and should not be used in pregnancy.

Pyridoxine should be given to all pregnant women receiving TB therapy to prevent peripheral neuropathy from isoniazid. Because many of the medications used to treat multidrug-resistant TB either are known to cause fetal abnormalities or have not been studied adequately, women of child-bearing age with multidrug-resistant TB should be advised to use birth control.

Breastfeeding

The first line antituberculous drugs cross into breast milk in variable amounts. Rifampicin is excreted into breast milk with milk to plasma ratio of 0.2. The amount transferred to the infant (0.05% of maternal dose) does not cause adverse effects. Pyrazinamide excretion into breast milk is minimal. With a maximum of 0.3% of the ingested dose reaching the infant. Streptomycin is excreted into breast milk with milk to plasma ratio of 0.5 to 1.0.94. Since the drug is very poorly absorbed orally, no significant absorption by the infant is to be expected from this. Ethambutol is secreted into breast milk with approximate milk to serum ratio of 1. The small concentrations of antituberculosis drugs in breast milk are not toxic to the newborn. Therefore breastfeeding should not be discouraged in HIV-seronegative women.[8] To minimise the level of anti-tuberculous drugs in the newborn, the mother can take her anti-tuberculous drugs immediately after a feed and substitute a bottle for the next feed, then go back to her usual feeding pattern until the next day.[12] However, breastfeeding is not recommended for HIV-infected women.

Children

Because of the high risk of disseminated tuberculosis in infants and children younger than 4 years of age, treatment should be started as soon as the diagnosis of tuberculosis is suspected. In general, the regimens recommended for adults are also the regimens of choice for infants, children, and adolescents with tuberculosis; with the exception that ethambutol is not used routinely in children. Because there is a lower bacillary burden in childhood-type tuberculosis there is less concern with the development of acquired drug resistance. However, children and adolescents may develop "adult-type" tuberculosis with upper lobe infiltration, cavitation, and sputum production. In such situations an initial phase of four drugs should be given until susceptibility is proven. When clinical or epidemiologic circumstances suggest an increased probability of INH resistance, EMB can be used safely at a dose of 15-20 mg/kg per day, even in children too young for routine eye testing. Streptomycin, kanamycin, or amikacin also can be used as the fourth drug, when necessary.

In cases of suspected drug-resistant tuberculosis in a child or when a source case isolate is not available, specimens for microbiological evaluation should be obtained via early morning gastric aspiration, bronchoalveolar lavage, or biopsy.

In general, extrapulmonary tuberculosis in children can be treated with the same regimens as pulmonary disease. Exceptions are disseminated tuberculosis and tuberculous meningitis, for which there are inadequate data to support 6-month therapy; thus 9-12 months of treatment is recommended.[13]

HIV Infection

The interaction between HIV and *M. tuberculosis* infection is bidirectional. Of HIV-infected individuals with pre-existing latent tuberculosis infection, 1-7 per cent will develop tuberculosis each year—a risk that is 4 to 25 times higher than the risk for those without HIV infection. HIV-infected patients who become newly infected with *M. tuberculosis* are also much more likely to develop symptomatic primary infection. Tuberculosis also has an impact on the course of HIV infection. In vitro, cytokines released in response to *M. tuberculosis* infection enhance HIV replication. HIV-infected patients with tuberculosis in developing countries develop more opportunistic infections than developed by patients who are at a similar stage of HIV infection but do not have tuberculosis.[8]

The clinical presentation is influenced by the patient's degree of immunosuppression and whether the tuberculosis has arisen from recently acquired infection or the reactivation of latent infection. Patients with relatively well-preserved immunity and pre-existing latent tuberculosis infection usually present with pulmonary tuberculosis and manifest the typical clinical, radiological and microbiological findings. In contrast, HIV-infected patients with primary tuberculosis and those with reactivated tuberculosis and impaired immunity (a CD_4 cell count of less than 200 per microlitre) often have atypical manifestations or pulmonary tuberculosis or present with extra-pulmonary or disseminated tuberculosis. Radiological features of pulmonary tuberculosis in these patients include the absence of cavitation, infiltrates in the mid and lower zones, and hilar lymphadenopathy.

The interpretation of the tuberculin skin test is complicated by the decline in cell-mediated immunity that accompanies HIV infection. For this reason, and because the risk of progression from latent to active tuberculosis infection is so high in HIV-infected people, a Mantoux test reaction of 5 mm or greater is considered to indicate infection with *M. tuberculosis*. This cut-off can be raised to 10 mm for patients with a CD_4 cell count greater than 500 per microlitre and a past history of BCG vaccination.

The treatment of tuberculosis in an HIV-infected patient is no straightforward, chiefly as a result of the complex interactions between anti-retroviral, anti-tuberculous and other drugs. Rifampicin is a potent inducer of hepatic cytochrome P_{450} 3A4 enzymes, while rifabutin is less so. The protease inhibitors and delavirdine are cytochrome P_{450} 3A4 inhibitors, nevirapine is an inducer, and efavirenz exerts mixed effects.

The occasional patient not being treated with anti-retroviral agents should undergo a standard treatment regimen of isoniazid, Rifampicin, pyrazinamide and ethambutol. Drugs in combination with anti-retroviral treatment, isoniazid, ethambutol and pyrazinamide are used in standard doses. Rifambutin is used instead of rifampicin, at a reduced dose of 150 milligrams daily with indinavir, nelfinavir and saquinavir soft-gel capsules, and at a dose of 450 milligrams daily with efavirenz.

Rifampicin is not generally recommended, although preliminary evidence suggests it may be possible to use with efavirenz or with ritonavir plus saquinavir.

Treatment duration is six months [2(HERZ)$_3$ 4 (HR)$_3$], unless the clinical or microbiological response is delayed, in which case treatment should be continued for at lest four months after sputum becomes culture negative.[14]

Diabetes

The patients with diabetes mellitus are at higher risk for the development of tuberculosis.[15,16] The prevalence of tuberculosis is greater in young, in those with low body mass index, in insulin dependent diabetes mellitus patients compared to those with non-insulin dependent diabetes mellitus patients, and in those with poorly controlled diabetes mellitus.[16] Patients with diabetes mellitus and coexistent tuberculosis have higher sputum positivity. However, the clinical symptoms and presentation of pulmonary tuberculosis are similar in diabetic and non-diabetic patients.

Increased susceptibility of patients with diabetes mellitus to tuberculosis could be due to neutrophilic dysfunction and impaired cytokines production.[17] Increased susceptibility to tuberculosis could also be due to thickened alveolar epithelium and pulmonary basal lamina, reduced pulmonary diffusion capacity, reduce lung volume and elastic recoil in patients with diabetes mellitus. The side effects of modern anti-tuberculosis treatment do not differ in with and without diabetes mellitus, except peripheral neuropathy which is much more common in patients of diabetes mellitus.[18]

On the other hand, the incidence of diabetes mellitus in pulmonary tuberculosis is not much higher than that in general population.[18] Further there is no specific radiological picture diagnostic of diabetic tuberculosis, except a predominance of exudative lesions in upper and mid zones.[18] Parahiler and lower zone involvement may or may not be there.

GERIATRIC

Tuberculosis exists as one of the top five killers in geriatric age group. The predisposing factors for its causation are poverty, inadequate housing, social neglect and a lack of awareness. It is often recognized late in the elderly. The occurrence of pulmonary tuberculosis is significantly higher than extrapulmonary tuberculosis in geriatric age group as compared to the younger age group. The Treatment outcomes of new smear-positive geriatric tuberculosis patients in comparison to younger tuberculosis patients showed significantly lower sputum conversion and cure rates, significantly higher exclusion rates from DOTS and relatively higher default and treatment failure rates.

REFERENCES

1. Sherlock S. Liver disease due to drugs. In drug induced disease. Associated Scientific Publishers, Amsterdam 1972;4:241.
2. Citron K.M. Tuberculosis chemotherapy. BMJ 1972;1:426.
3. Segarra PV, Lorain V, Sherman D.S. Ethambutol treatment of tuberculosis in a controlled trial. Scand J. Resp Dis 1968;49:202.
4. Smith JP, Scharer L. Serum transaminase elevation and other hepatic abnormalities in patients receiving isoniazid. Ann. Inter. Med. 1969; 71:1113.
5. Byrd RB, Nelson R, Elliot RC Isoniazid toxicity. JAMA 1972;220:1471.
6. Lal S, Singhal SN Burley DN. Crossley G. Effect of Rifampicin and isoniazid on liver function. BMJ 1972;1:148.
7. Less AW Toxicity in newly diagnosed cases of pulmonary tuberculosis treated with ethionamide. Am. Rev. Resp. Dis. 1972;106:357.
8. Management, control and prevention of tuberculosis, *Guidelines for Health Care Providers (2002-2005)*, Department of Human Services, Victorian Government Department of Human Services, Melbourne Victoria.
9. Parathasarathy R, Sarma UR, Janardhanan B *et al.* Hepatic toxicity in South Indian patients during treatment of tuberculosis with short course regimens containing INH, RMP and PZA. Tubercle 1986;67:99-108.
10. Carter EJ and Mates S. 'Tuberculosis during pregnancy. The Rhode Island Experience, 1987-1991', *Chest* 1994;106:1466-70.
11. Potworowska M, Sianozecka F, Szufladwicz R. Ethionamide treatment and pregnancy. Pol Med J. 1966; 5:1152-1158.
12. Management, Control and Prevention of Tuberculosis *Guidelines for Health Care Providers (2002-2005)* Published by Rural and Regional Health and Aged Care Services Division, Victorian Government Department of Human Services, Melbourne Victoria. August 2002.
13. Treatment of Tuberculosis, American Thoracic Society, CDC, and Infectious Diseases Society of America, June 20, 2003/52(RR11);1-77.

14. Burman, W and Jones, B. 'Treatment of HIV-related tuberculosis in the era of effective anti-retro viral therapy'. Am J Respir Crit Care Med 2001;164:7-12.
15. Lester FT. Clinical features complications and mortality in type 1 diabetes mellitus in Addis Ababa-1990. QJM 1992;83:389-99.
16. Swai AB, Mclarty DG. Mugusi F. Tuberculosis in diabetic patients in Tanzania. Trop Doct 990;20:147-50.
17. Uno K. Nakano K. Maruo N. Onodera H. Meta H, Kurosu I, Akatani K. Determination of interferon-alpha-producing capacity in whole blood culture from patients with various disease and from healthy persons. J interferon cytokine Res. 1996;16:911-18.
18. Jain NK. Madan A. Sharma TN, Purohit SD. Agrawal K. Agnihotri S, Durlabhji P. Kala D. Diabetic Tuberculosis; A changing pattern. Lung India 1985; III No. 1:11-14.

Chapter nineteen

Multi-Drug Resistant Tuberculosis

BL Bhardwaj, RS Bhatia

Any discussion on tuberculosis starts with figures which tend to numb the mind. About one third of the world's population is infected by mycobacterium tuberculosis. Deaths from tuberculosis comprise 25% of all avoidable deaths in developing countries. 95% of tuberculosis cases and 98% of tuberculosis[6] deaths are in developing countries; 75% of these are in the economically productive age group. In India, > 20000 people become infected and > 5000 develop the disease daily. 'One patient dies every minute.' India has the highest number of tuberculosis cases for any country in the world and many of these are Multidrug Resistant (MDR). WHO and IUATLD has identified certain 'Hot Zones' i.e. areas with > 3% MDR Tuberculosis and India is one of them. Various surveys have been done to estimate the problem. M. tuberculosis isolates in Indore showed MDR @ 8.1%. In Jodhpur, sputum samples of pulmonary tuberculosis cases tested for sensitivity showed primary MDR as 3.3% and acquired MDR as 3.8.2%. In Delhi, incidence of MDR-TB was found to be 14%.

DRUG RESISTANCE

It is defined as temporary or permanent capacity of an organism and their progeny to remain viable or to multiply in the presence of that particular concentration of a drug which would normally destroy or inhibit the growth of other similar cells.

DRUG RESISTANT TUBERCULOSIS

This is a case of tuberculosis (usually pulmonary) excreting bacilli resistant to one or more antituberculosis drugs. It is said to be of the following types:

1. Primary Resistance

It is the bacterial resistance in patients who have certainly not had any prior treatment with antituberculosis drugs (ATT).

2. Initial Resistance

After clinical assessment, if it is doubtful that the patient really has not received prior ATT, then it is called initial resistance. It may be primary resistance or it may be undisclosed acquired resistance.

3. Acquired Resistance

In patients with some record of previous ATT, the bacterial resistance is called acquired resistance.

The occurrence of primary resistance is a consequence of the level of acquired resistance in the community. The greater the number of patients who are excretors of resistant bacilli during or after treatment, the higher the risk of transmission of resistant bacilli to healthy individuals and of emergence of new cases with primary resistance. Primary and acquired resistance differ in terms of their prevalence and severity in the following ways:

1. The rate of primary resistance is lower than the rate of acquired resistance.
2. Primary resistance is less severe than acquired resistance:
   - Primary resistance is more often to one drug (streptomycin or isoniazid) than to two drugs. Primary resistance to three or more drugs or primary MDR is exceptional. By contrast, acquired resistance usually concerns two drugs or more and MDR is relatively frequent.
   - The level of resistance (i.e. the minimum inhibitory concentration of antibiotics) is lower in primary than in acquired resistance.

This is why primary resistance hardly affects the outcome of treatment with standard regimens combining four drugs in the initial phase of treatment in new smear positive patients.

FAILURE OF RETREATMENT

It is a tuberculosis patient excreting bacilli either after 5 months, or after completion of the 8-month retreatment regimen (RTR), given under direct supervision. This RTR consists of 3 drugs throughout (isoniazid (H), rifampicin (R), ethambutol (E) supplemented by pyrazinamide (Z) during the first 3 months and streptomycin (S) during the first 2 months. These cases are usually resistant to at least one or two of the main bactericidal drugs given (H and/or R). These are also called 'chronic cases' when they have received at least two courses of chemotherapy including one failure of RTR. These cases are usually excretors of resistant bacilli and often of MDR bacilli.

MULTIDRUG RESISTANT TUBERCULOSIS

It is the type of drug resistance where tuberculosis bacilli are resistant to both isoniazid and rifampicin. It is the most severe form of bacterial resistance. Usually MDR tuberculosis occurs in chronic cases and represents a significant proportion of tuberculosis patients with acquired resistance. Exceptionally, MDR tuberculosis is observed in new cases.

MECHANISM OF DRUG RESISTANCE

Drug resistance occurs in mycobacterium tuberculosis by a random, single step, spontaneous mutation occurring at a low but predictable frequency (estimated to be 1 in 10^8 for R, 10^6 for H and 10^5 for S, E, PAS, Ethionamide, Cycloserine and thiacetazone. For resistance to both H and R, the frequency is very less, 1 in 10^14 (i.e. 10^8 × 10^6). So, in lesions with more bacillary load e.g. cavitary disease, the rate of occurrence of resistance is high.

Virtually all isolates resistant to R have a mutation in rpoB gene that alters the sequence of a 27 AA region of β subunit of RNA polymerase, so that R cannot bind and target bacterial RNA polymerase.

INH resistant bacilli have mutations in katG gene encoding catalase peroxidase which transforms INH into active form for intracellular action. Other genes implicated in INH resistance are inhA (encoding an enzyme involved in cell wall synthesis), ahpC (encoding an enzyme component of antioxidant reductase) and kasA genes.

W strain of mycobacterium tuberculosis (resistance to H, E, R and S) has a characteristic IS6110 restriction fragment length polymorphism banding pattern.

Similarly, resistance to other drugs is due to various mutations e.g. S resistance associated with mutation on rrs and rpsL gene; Z resistance with pncA gene; E resistance with embB gene (60%); fluoroquinolone resistance with gyrA gene and kanamycin resistance with rrs gene. Several other new alleles as molecular genetic basis of drug resistance have also been identified.

MDR strains arise by serial sequential accumulation or selection of resistant mutants for individual drugs.

THE GENESIS OF MDR TUBERCULOSIS

As with other forms of drug resistance, the phenomenon of MDR tuberculosis is entirely MAN-MADE. Drug resistant bacilli are the consequence of human error in any of the following:

1. *Prescription of chemotherapy.* The most common errors are:
   - The prescription of inadequate chemotherapy to multibacillary pulmonary tuberculosis.
   - The addition of one extra drug in case of failure, and repeating the addition of a further drug when the patient relapses after what amounts to monotherapy.
2. *Management of drug supply.* The most common errors are:
   - The difficulty experienced by poor patients in obtaining all the drugs that they need due to lack of financial resources.
   - Frequent or prolonged shortages of antituberculosis drugs.
   - Use of drugs or drug combinations of unproven bioavailability.

3. *Case management.* The following also have the effect of multiplying the risk of successive monotherapies and selection of resistant bacilli:
   - The patient's lack of knowledge due to lack of information or inadequate explanation before starting treatment.
   - The lack of direct supervision of treatment especially during the initial phase.

HIV per se is not a risk factor for development of MDR Tuberculosis, but the increased incidence of MDR in HIV positive patients may be related to prior treatment.

LAB DIAGNOSIS

The following methods can be used:

1. *Culture and sensitivity:* This can be done with the help of either 7 H10 or 7H11 Middlebrook or Lowenstein-Jensen media. It requires 12-16 weeks, leading to delay in the initiation of treatment.
2. *Direct sensitivity test:* Done without culturing by directly inoculating drug in the medium. It saves 4 weeks.
3. *Slide culture test:* It is a simple test. Gives results in 8-10 days.
4. *BACTEC System:* It is a radiometric method of measuring radioactive CO_2, a product of bacterial metabolisms. Results available in 10-14 days.
5. *Luciferase reporter mycobacteriophage (LRP) test:* It is a very sensitive and specific test. Report available in 18-72 hours.
6. *Polymerase chain reaction (PCR) test:* Done using single stranded confirmation polymorphism and line probe assays. Results within 24 hours.
7. *Restriction fragment length polymorphism:* Use of DNA probes is done. It is also successful in epidemiological studies in outbreak of tuberculosis.
8. Other methods include e.g. High performance liquid chromatography, Pulse field gel electrophoresis and Ligand chain reaction assays etc.

BASIC PRINCIPLES FOR MANAGEMENT OF MDR TUBERCULOSIS

Prevention

Even if the proportion of MDR tuberculosis is high, the top priority is not the management, but the prevention of MDR tuberculosis; because, a poor program can generate MDR tuberculosis much faster than any program can cure it. With good treatment meticulously prescribed and administered, MDR tuberculosis should not occur. So, concentration should be on ensuring that all new patients are cured by completing the standard treatment as follows:

1. **In New Cases:** The best prevention is to give each new case of sputum positive pulmonary tuberculosis an effective short course ATT i.e. 6-8 months with at least 2 months of HRZ + E/S given under direct observation/

supervision. WHO recommended regimens are as effective in patients with bacilli initially resistant to H and/or S as in patients with susceptible bacilli.

2. **In Old Cases:** In this group of patients, 3 subpopulations can be observed:
   - Patients excreting bacilli still susceptible to all ATT drugs.
   - Patients excreting bacilli resistant to at least H, but still susceptible to R.
   - Patients excreting bacilli resistant to at least H and R.

In patients who have failed after the first course of ATT, the proportion of people excreting bacilli still susceptible to all drugs is usually higher than the proportion of the two other subpopulations. The standard WHO can cure majority of these patients.

In patients who have failed RTR, the proportion of patients excreting resistant bacilli is the majority (upto 80%) and MDR tuberculosis can be as high as 50% of this. For this reason, a second application of RTR is likely to fail.

ASSESSING THE CASE OF APPARENT MDR TUBERCULOSIS

The suspicion of MDR tuberculosis occurs in two situations:

A. When a report of MDR tuberculosis strains from a laboratory is received.

B. When a smear positive patient shows no response to the standard RTR.

SOME PROVISOS

- Apparent MDR strains reported by a local lab should not be taken uncritically at face value. If the result is a single one and if it does not accord with clinical data, it should be discussed with the bacteriologist (if possible) and at least one, preferably two sets, should be repeated.
- It is to be remembered that many apparent treatment failures are due to the patient having failed to take his treatment and not due to MDR bacilli. Such patients should respond to the standard fully supervised RTR.
- Just because the patient is registered in a standard national regimen, it should not be assumed that the patient has necessarily received it. Checking with the records, the patient, the patient's family and the previous doctor is required. There may well have been errors. Careful notes from these documents of the dose of each drug, its frequency of administration and the dates when each drug was started and stopped should be made.
- The criteria of RTR failure are mainly bacteriological. But not all positive bacteriological results necessarily mean failure.

A. Persistently Sputum Positive

- If the patient is still sputum positive after 2-3 months of RTR, it should be checked carefully whether he has taken all the drugs as prescribed. This is the most common cause of failure. However, some patients with severe disease may take longer to convert from sputum positive to negative. Its no use rushing into changing treatment. If the number of bacilli in direct smear is less and he is improving clinically and radiologically, this is particularly reassuring.

- Persistent positivity at 5-6 months makes genuine treatment failure much more likely. Again the most common cause is failure to take drugs. But if it is certain that the patient is taking the drugs, it is highly probable that the bacilli are resistant to all the drugs he is receiving. Checking the apparent persistent positivity by further sputum smears and culture is required.
- Fall and rise phenomenon
  Sputum smear initially becomes negative (or even less positive), and then later becomes persistently positive. This indicates failure either due to the patient having ceased to take drugs or sometimes to the resistance to all the drugs. In the latter case, the fall is due to initial decrease in the number of bacilli and the rise later on due to the selective growth of resistant bacilli.

B. Radiological Deterioration

This may be a sign of failure but may also be due to intercurrent pneumonia or pulmonary embolism or supervening carcinoma. If it is not accompanied by bacteriological deterioration, it is less likely to be due to tuberculosis. Chest X-ray should be repeated after 2-3 weeks.

C. Clinical Deterioration

This is the least reliable evidence of failure.

AVAILABLE ANTI-TUBERCULAR DRUGS

Standard essential anti-tuberculosis drugs

Drug	*Activity*	*Brief Description*
Isoniazid Low 5 mg/kg/d High 10-15 mg/kg/d	Bactericidal (active) and Static (Resting). Ag both intra and extra cell	S/E Hepatitis, Peripheral Neuropathy, rash, fever. Give pyridoxine 150 mg daily.
Rifampicin 10 mg/kg/d	Bactericidal (both intra and extra cell)	S/E GI upset, Hepatitis, Rash, Haemolytic anaemia, Thrombocytopenia, orange, secretions. Important enzyme inducer.
Pyrazinamide 15-30 mg/kg/d	Bactericidal in acid pH	Resistance neither easy to acquire nor easy to prove by sensitivity tests. S/E Hepatotoxicity, H^uricemia, polyarthralgias.
Ethambutol 15 mg/kg/d	Bacterio Static	Useless for treatment of MDR TB; but if bacilli sensitive, then may be given as companion drug to prevent resistance to other drugs. S/E retrobulbar neuritis.

Contd.

Contd.

Thiacetazone 150 mg tid	Bacterio Static	No place in MDR except as last resort. Cross resistance and toxicity with thio-amides. S/E hepatotoxicity, BM suppression and cutaneous reactions (in HIV).
Streptomycin 0.75-1 gm daily	Bactericidal (rapidly dividing extracell org)	Poor penetration into meninges. Resistance less common now since wider use of Emb and use limited to initial 2 months. S/E ototoxicity, Nephrotoxicity and NM blockade. Not used in pregnancy and renal insufficiency.

SECOND LINE ANTI-TUBERCULOSIS DRUGS

Drug	*Activity*	*Brief Description*
Aminoglycoside Kanamycin (0.75-1 gm/d) Amikacin (0.5-0.75 gm/d) Capreomycin (0.75-1 gm/d)	Bactericidal against actively multiplying organisms	Kana least and Capreo most expensive. Complete cross resistance between Kana and Amika. Bacilli res to both still susceptible to Capreo. Inj Kana and Capreo painful. S/E Ototoxicity and Nephrotoxicity. Deafness less with Capreo. Not used in pregnancy. Avoided in children.
Thioamides Ethionamide (0.75-1 gm/d Prothionamide (0.75-1 g/d)	Bacterio static	Complete cross resistance between them. 70% strains res to these are resistant to Th but not vice versa. S/E N and V, anorexia, abd discomfort. Give with milk at bed time. No in pregnancy.
Fluoroquinolones Ofloxacin (400 mg bd) Ciprofloxacin (750 mg bd) Suprafloxacin (200-400 mg bd) Levofloxacin (500 mg od) Gatifloxacin (400 mg od) Moxifloxacin	Bactericidal (low)	Complete cross resistance within the group. Useful with other drugs. S/E N and V, anorexia, dizziness, mood changes, ARF. Sparflox may induce ↑QT interval and photosensitivity
Cycloserine (0.75-1 gm/d) and Terizodone)	Bacterio static	Complete cross resistance, none with others. So, valuable to prevent resistance to other drugs. Highly toxic. S/E mainly related to CNS. May lead to convulsions and suicidal tendencies. Pyridoxine and tranquilizers may help.

Contd.

Contd.

PAS (4 gm tid)	Bacterio static	Valuable for preventing resistance to other bactericidals. Bulky and unpleasant because of GI discomfort. Has antithyroid effect.

Other drugs

- Rifabutin (150 mg/d)—Similar to Rifampicin. Inhibits a quarter of R res strains. Recommended over R in HIV.
- Clarithromycin (500 mg bd)—Highly concentrated in macrophages. S/E N and V, hepatitis. Dose ↓ in renal failure.
- Rifapentine, Clofazimine and Amoxi-clav—Not much role in MDR tuberculosis.

DESIGNING A CHEMOTHERAPY REGIMEN FOR THE PATIENT

Susceptibility testing is not recommended for all new cases since it is not practicable and is expensive. It is recommended either in representative samples as an epidemiological tool for monitoring bacterial resistance in a region or in suspected drug resistant patients. Culture and reliable tests for drug resistance to standard essential drugs and also to second line drugs should be carried out.

Patients with resistance to H and additional resistance, or suspected resistance, to S and/or Th (but not R) should respond well to the standard RTR.

Patients considered failure of RTR and those who have a variety of non standard bad regimens will often require at least some second line drugs.

Treatment of patients with MDR tuberculosis has to involve second line reserve drugs other than the essential ATT drugs i.e. R, H, Z, E, S and Th. The reserve drugs are much more expensive, less effective and have many more side effects than the essential drugs. So, their use should be limited in order to prevent the emergence of incurable tuberculosis.

It must be made clear to the patient and staff that meticulously taking the prescribed reserve regimen is all that stands between the patient and death. The patient must try to tolerate any unpleasant side effects in order to achieve survival. He must remain under direct observation, with each dose supervised, at least until the sputum is negative. He must get permanent psychological support.

In designing a regimen, *the aim should not be to keep drugs in reserve.* That is the best way to lose one battle after another. As outlined above, it should be decided to what drugs the patients bacilli are (or are likely to be) still sensitive. Then, the regimen likely to be most effective for him should be prescribed.

Designing an appropriate regimen for the individual patient needs experience, skill, allocation of time and patience to define precisely the following:

1. Which regimen(s) the patient has received previously.
2. Whether the patient took all the drugs in each regimen prescribed and for how long.

3. To find out what happened bacteriologically, in terms of sputum positivity (at least by direct smear, if not culture) during and after the administration of each regimen. Clinical and radiological progress or deterioration is much less reliable, but may be used as a check on the bacteriological results.

In the first place drugs which the patient has not had previously should be prescribed. The bacilli are fairly certain to be sensitive to these. The practice of adding H to these drugs confers no advantage. If there is evidence to suggest that the bacilli remain sensitive to an essential drug, in spite of the patient having received it in an unreliable combination, it may be *added* to the regimen but it is not to be relied upon to prevent further resistance.

Consideration of cross resistance between drugs is very important for MDR Tuberculosis because it is ineffective to combine two drugs of the same group and to combine a drug potentially ineffective because of cross resistance.

The initial regimen should consist of at least three drugs, preferably 4-5, to which the bacilli are likely to be fully sensitive. Among these drugs, it is desirable to use in combination an injectable aminoglycoside and Z (even if previously used because resistance is usually unlikely). The combination has a good bactericidal activity. When the sputum has converted to negative, one or more weaker drugs causing side effects may be withdrawn. The treatment with these regimens should be continued for at least 18 months after sputum conversion to prevent relapse. In case of resistance to most of the first line drugs, treatment should continue for at least 24 months.

In any regimen chosen, the treatment should be given daily and should be directly observed. It is also mandatory to monitor bacteriological results (smear and culture) monthly from the second month until the sixth month and then quarterly until the end of treatment.

SPECIAL CLINICAL SITUATIONS

In renal failure, aminoglycosides not given and ethambutol given only if serum levels can be monitored. In severe cases, dose of H and Z may have to be reduced. In pregnancy, all 4 standard essential ATT drugs can be used, but close liver function monitoring is recommended. ATT not a contraindication to breast feeding. Silicotuberculosis necessitates extension of ATT by two months. In hepatic disease H and R given under close monitoring, but Z should be avoided. Treatment in skeletal, meningeal and miliary tuberculosis needs to be extended.

SOME EXAMPLES OF ACCEPTABLE REGIMENS

A delay of 2-4 months is usual in obtaining susceptibility results. So, in practice, two situations should be considered:

A. SUSCEPTIBILITY TEST RESULTS NOT AVAILABLE

A new regimen should be initiated in which at least 3 drugs never used and Z should be used. After sputum conversion (usually 3-4 months), two drugs more active and best tolerated should be employed in continuation phase.

Initial phase		*Continuation phase*	
Drugs	*Minimum duration*	*Drugs*	*Duration*
1. Aminoglycoside 2. Ethionamide 3. Pyrazinamide 4. Quinolone*	3 months or till sputum conversion	1. Ethionamide 2. Quinolone	18 months after sputum conversion

* If not tolerated, may use cycloserine/PAS.

B. SUSCEPTIBILITY TEST RESULTS AVAILABLE

Drug resistant to INH, but susceptible to rifampicin

Resistance to	*Initial phase*		*Continuation phase*	
	Drugs	*Minimum duration*	*Drugs*	*Duration*
Isoniazid (streptomycin, thiacetazone)	1. Rifampicin 2. Aminoglycosides 3. Pyrazinamide 4. Ethambutol	2-3 months or till sputum conversion	1. Rifampicin 2. Ethambutol	6 months after sputum conversion
Isoniazid and ethambutol/ Streptomycin	1. Rifampicin 2. Aminoglycosides 3. Pyrazinamide 4. Ethionamide*	3 months or till sputum conversion	1. Rifampicin 2. Ethionamide*	6 months after sputum conversion

* If ethionamide not available or poorly tolerated even at 500 mg, use quinolone.

Multidrug resistant

Resistance to	*Initial phase*		*Continuation phase*	
	Drugs	*Minimum duration*	*Drugs*	*Duration*
Isoniazid and rifampicin	1. Aminoglycosides 2. Ethionamide 3. Pyrazinamide* 4. Quinolone 5. Ethambutol	3 months or till sputum conversion	1. Ethionamide 2. Quinolone 3. Ehtambutol	18 months after sputum conversion
Isoniazid rifampicin streptomycin and ethambutol	1. Aminoglycosides 2. Ethionamide 3. Pyrazinamide 4. Quinolone 5. Cycloserine/PAS	3 months or till sputum conversion	1. Ethionamide 2. Quinolone 3. Cycloserine/ PAS	18 months after sputum conversion

* If resistance to pyrazinamide duly proven, then add cycloserine/PAS.

Note: In MDR meningitis, alternate day intrathecal levofloxacin and Amikacin with high dose H, E and Z can be used.

NEWER APPROACHES IN THE MANAGEMENT

Surgery should be considered for a patient with bacilli resistant to all except 2-3 relatively weaker drugs. Unfortunately many such patients have too extensive disease and/or too poor lung function for surgery to be possible. If the patient has a large localised cavity with little other disease, reasonable lung function and only 2-3 weak drugs available, surgery should be seriously considered. To avoid complications, operate when the bacillary population is likely to be at its lowest. Experience has shown that most favourable time is after 2 months' ATT. After surgery, same regimen should be continued for at least 18 months.

Laser therapy (with CO_2, YAG, He and Ne) acts by decreasing bacillary load in moderately advanced disease and increases penetration of drugs in walled off lesions. It is also valuable in management of tracheal/bronchial stenosis.

Addition of immunotherapy with M. vaccae has shown to improve rate of cure, especially in patients with short disease, but multiple dosing can have beneficial effects in chronic patients. Immunomodulators like γ-interferon, TNF, Interleukin-2 and levamisole in complicated cases may prove to be useful.

Treatment of MDR TB by non-antibiotics like phenothiazines offers great potential. These drugs are concentrated in macrophages and they exert their effects on the bacterial inner membrane. Experimental trials with surfactant (Myramistine) confirmed that it enhanced the sensitivity of MDR strains to ATT.

'Suicide gene' which involves the use of a genetic manipulation to restore sensitivity to a drug is another novel approach.

DOTS-PLUS

Since the presence of MDR tuberculosis signals tuberculosis program failure, the key to global tuberculosis control remains the adoption of a 'DOTS-Plus' programme. In 1999, WHO established the Working Group on DOTS-Plus for MDR tuberculosis. DOTS-Plus is a comprehensive management strategy under development and testing. DOTS-Plus takes into account specific issues (such as the use of second-line anti-TB drugs) that need to be addressed in areas where there is high prevalence of MDR-TB. Thus, DOTS-Plus works as a supplement to the standard DOTS strategy. DOTS-Plus is not intended as a universal strategy, and is not required in all settings. DOTS-Plus should be implemented in selected areas with moderate to high levels of MDR-TB in order to combat an emerging epidemic. It is best initiated in settings where DOTS implementation is proper. It requires specialized clinical expertise, a surveillance component, high quality lab support, and uninterrupted but regulated supply of 2nd line drugs and adequate delivery resources. DOTS-Plus has not yet been implemented in India.

REFERENCES

1. Crofton John, Chaulet Pierre, Maher Dermott; Guidelines for the management of drug resistant tuberculosis. WHO/TB/96/210, 1997.
2. Chatterji RS; Multidrug resistance in tuberculosis. Medicine update, 2004;14:246-54.
3. Narain JP; Multidrug resistant tuberculosis. Tuberculosis epidemiology and control (WHO#SEA/TB/248), 2002;105-115.
4. O'Brien RJ, Raviglione MC; Tuberculosis. Harrison's Principles of Internal Medicine, 16th Ed, 953-966.
5. Di PerriG, Bonora S; which agents should we use for the treatment of MDR-Mycobacterium tuberculosis, J. Antimicrob. Chemother; 2004;54:593-602.

Chapter twenty

Revised National Tuberculosis Control Programme

Jai Kishan

National Tuberculosis Control Program (NTP) was designed by National Tuberculosis Institute, Bangalore on the sound technical principles of case finding and treatment in the year 1962. NTP was integrated with general health service with District TB Centre (DTC) as a nodal center under NTP. Despite the fact that same principles of diagnosis and treatment were available under NTP as with the developed countries yet it failed in India. Main causes of failure of NTP were greater emphasis on diagnosis by X-ray and not by smear examination, less emphasis on potentially infectious cases in the community, apathy of health workers, erratic drug supply, improper supervision and follow up led to high default rates. Only 1/3rd of patient on long term and 1/2 patients on short course chemotherapy completed treatment. District TB officer was not able to supervise the vast area of the whole district. Reporting from DTC's to NTI was not proper. DOTS is internationally recommended strategy to ensure cure of tuberculosis. Based on the above findings the shortcomings of NTP were removed and its strengths in corporated, the revised national tuberculosis control program (RNTCP) with 5 components was formulated.

i. *Political and administrative commitment:* In order to get funding for regular supply of drugs, staffing and to get support from all the agencies required for program. There was creation of tuberculosis unit for a population of 5 lakhs with Medical Officer TB Control, Senior Treatment Supervisor, and Senior Tuberculosis Laboratory Supervisor for proper and comprehensive supervision.

ii. *Good quality diagnosis by sputum smear examination:* By creating designated microscopy center at a population of one lakh and provision of good quality binocular Microscopes and regular supply of quality reagents. There is a system of gradation of sputum and cross checking by STLS for maintaining quality of sputum smear examination. Laboratory Technicians are also given training under the RNTCP thereby laying stress on diagnosis of smear positive cases by sputum smear examination who are a potential threat for spread of tuberculosis in the community. If a sputum smear positive patient is not given treatment then he is likely to transmit infection to 10-15 persons in a year. Under the RNTCP case finding is amongst symptomatics attending the health centers. According to a study by Anderson and Banerjee majority of the patients of sputum positive pulmonary tuberculosis contact the health centers prompted by the symptoms of cough, expectoration, fever, pain chest or haemoptysis. Under RNTCP no active case findings are undertaken. Any patients have symptoms of cough of more than 3 weeks with or without other symptoms or pulmonary tuberculosis is subjected to 3 sputum specimens examinations (1st Spot, 2nd early morning specimen and 3rd spot) in two days. Two sputum smear examinations could detect more than 89% cases in a study at NTI Bangalore and yield of 1st, 2nd and 3rd sputum smear examination was 83.4%, 95.6% and 100% in a study in Tanzania and 83%, 96% and 100% in a study at Malawi. Examination of 3 sputum smear examination in ideal as per WHO. Sputum smear examination is cheap, readily available and highly specific for diagnosis of pulmonary tuberculosis amongst symptomatics attending chest clinics. Specificity is more than 98% and false positivity is only 1.3%-2.6%. Diagnosis by X-ray examination is having inherent disadvantage of laying stress on noninfectious cases and ignoring sputum positive cases. Interobserver variation in X-ray reading is 40% and intraobserver variation in X-ray reading for tuberculosis is 20%. Based on X-ray examination vast majority of cases may be started on antituberculosis treatment unnecessarily. Sputum smear examination at 2M, 5M and at end of treatment is also effective in monitoring the progress of patents. Radiological changes alone for monitoring can be very misleading.

iii. *Good quality treatment and free regular supply of drugs* like NTP under RNTCP also the treatment of tuberculosis is home based. Hospitalisation under RNTCP is undertaken in case of complications, toxicity of drugs, very serious patients or under social compulsion where patient has got no family support. Domiciliary treatment is as effective as hospital treatment was proved beyond doubt in a study at Tuberculosis Research Center, Madras. In this study rest and diet were not found to have any role and chances of tuberculosis infection or disease was found to be essentially equal in the contact of sanatorium and home treatment cases. Whatever harm a patient could have done, is before starting treatment. A patient become relatively noninfectious within two weeks of start of effective chemotherapeutic regimen.

The reasons of failure of NTP were nonstandardized treatment prescribed by doctors and erratic drug supply. In a study conducted by Uplekar it was observed that 82 regimens were prescribed by 100 doctors for treatment of pulmonary tuberculosis. Under RNTCP all the patients depending upon their priority for treatment from the patient and public health point of view have been categorized into three catetories and now standardized treatment regimens are prescribed under RNTCP as in Table 20.1 given below.

Table 20.1: Category of patients and categories of treatment

Category of treatment	*Type of patient*	*Regimen**
Category I	New sputum smear-positive seriously ill sputum smear-negative seriously ill extra-pulmonary**	2 $(HRZE)_3$ 4 $(HR)_3$
Category II	Sputum smear-positive Relapse*** Sputum smear-positive Failure*** Sputum smear-positive Treatment after Default	2 $(HRZES)_3$ 1 $(HRZE)_3$ 5 $(HRE)_3$
Category III	Sputum smear-negative, extra-pulmonary, not seriously ill	2 $(HRZ)_3$ 4 $(HR)_3$

* The number before the letters refers to the number of months of treatment. The subscript after the letters refers to the number of doses per week. H: Isoniazid (600 mg), R Rifampicin (450 mg), Z: Pyrazinamide (1500 mg), E: Ethambutol (1200 mg), S: Streptomycin (750 mg). Patients who weigh more than 60 kg received additional rifampicin 150 mg. Patients more than 50 years old and those who weigh less than 30 kg receive streptomycin 500 mg. Patients in categories I and II who have a positive sputum smear at the end of the initial intensive phase receive an additional month of intensive phase treatment.

** Examples of seriously ill extra-pulmonary TB cases are meningitis, disseminated TB, tuberculosis pericarditis, peritonitis, bilateral or extensive pleurisy, spinal TB with neurological complications and intestinal and genitourinary TB.

*** In rare and exceptional cases, patients who are sputum smear-negative or who have extra-pulmonary disease can be Relapse or Failure. The diagnosis in all such cases should always be made by an MO and should be supported by culture or histological evidence of current, active TB. In these cases, the patient should be categorized as "Other" and given Category II treatment.

A full course of 6 or 8 months has been packed in the boxes. A box of full course is earmarked for the patient while starting the treatment hence ensuring availability of drugs for full duration of treatment. There is central procurement of these drugs and quality of drugs is maintained by checking the quantity, quality and bioavailability of drugs. Proper storage of these drugs is undertaken to ensure potency of drugs. Monitoring of treatment response is underaken by doing follow up smear examination highly at end of intensive phase, two months of continuation phase at end of treatment. Patients found smear positive at end of intensive phase are given an additional one month of intensive phase for which ample quantity of extension pouches are available. In order to avoid stockout, a stock of 6 months is kept at district tuberculosis centers. Treatment outcome at the end of treatment is evaluated and reported. Under RNTCP intermittent treatment is given. Intermittent treatment is based on the principle of lag period. If the bacilli are subjected to the effective concentration of a drug then they are not able to grow for certain period in the drug free environment for certain period which is called as lag period.

Lag period for various drugs is given as in Table 20.2 given below.

Lag in growth of mycobacterium tuberculosis after temporary exposures to drugs.

Table 20.2

Drug	*Concentration (mg/litre)*	*Lag (days) after exposure for*
Isoniazid	1	6-9
Rifampicin	0.2	2-3
Pyrazinamide	50	40[b]
Ethambutol	10	4-5
Streptomycin	5	8-10
Ethionamide	5	10
Cycloserine	100	4-8
Thioacetazone	10	0

Doses of drugs in intermittent regimens is as in Table 20.3 given below:

Table 20.3

Drug	*Daily dosage, mg/kg (gange)*	*Doses of drugs*	
	Daily treatment	*Treatment three times a week*	*Treatment twice a week*[b]
Isoniazid	5 (4-6)	10 (8-12)	15 (13-17)
Rifampicin	10 (8-12)	10 (8-12)	10 (8-12)
Pyrazinamide	25 (20-30)	35 (30-40)	50 (40-60)
Streptomycin	15 (12-18)	15 (12-18)	15 (12-18)
Ethambutol	15 (13-17)	30 (25-35)	45 (40-50)
Thioacetazone	2.5 (2-3)	NA	NA

Chapter twenty-one

TB Eradication—Where We Stand

SS Arora, RS Bhatia

Tuberculosis is a leading public health problem worldwide particularly in the developing countries. In view of the seriousness of the problem, WHO in 1993 declared it to be a Global Emergency. Two million of these people die every year. These constitute 26% of eminently avoidable adult deaths worldwide. In South-East Asian Region, nearly 3 million cases and 700,000 deaths occur every year; five countries—Bangladesh, India, Indonesia, Myanmar and Thailand account for 95% of these deaths. This morbidity and mortality occur, mainly in the economically productive ages between 15-60 years, directly affecting the nations' economies. The situation is likely to be further complicated by the rapidly expanding HIV/AIDS epidemic and the emergence of multidrug resistance strains of TB.

Many cases remain undiagnosed, primarily due to the failure of health system to promptly diagnose and properly treat who seek care. Patients also require information on the use of TB drugs and the location of the diagnostic facilities. Of patients diagnosed, less than half, under previous programmes, completed treatment. Patients who do not complete treatment may then continue to infect others in the community. It is estimated that one infectious patient infects an average of 10-15 people. India's persistent problems of poverty, rapid population growth, increasing migration, and poor health infrastructure for implementation of national health programmes in the past have only added to the grim scenario. Patients who do not complete their treatment or who take treatment irregularly on account of inadequate prescribing, unreliable drug supplies, poor patient motivation, or financial and other reasons can develop Multidrug Resistant TB (MDR-TB). Multidrug Resistant TB is difficult, and very expensive to treat. HIV is an important risk factor for the development of tuberculosis. As a result, in many areas, a parallel epidemic of TB is following the AIDS pandemic. It is estimated that in the next 3-5 years, 20-25% of cases in some parts of the SEA Region could be directly attributed to HIV. HIV-associated TB is more difficult to diagnose, although response to short-course of treatment is equally good.

TB accounts for one third of AIDS deaths worldwide. It is the biggest killer of people who are HIV-positive. If you are HIV-positive, you are 30 times more likely to get sick with TB once infected. TB kills more women than all causes of maternal mortality put together. Over 100,000 children will die needlessly from TB this year. Drug-resistance can develop when patients get the wrong drugs, drug supply is unreliable or patients stop taking their medicines because they feel better. In countrties that are poor, MDR-TB that cannot be treated with standard medicines can be a death sentence. Eighty percent of TB victims are in the most economically productive years of their lives. The situation is likely to be further complicated with the rapid spread of HIV and emergence of drug resistant strains in the region. Nearly 60% of AIDS cases develop TB indicating that the latter is the most common life threatening opportunistic infection associated with HIV.

Traditionally, provision of TB treatment services has been the most common area for collaboration. However, with the advent of DOTS, NGO participation in stopping TB has taken on even greater importance. Being closer to the communities they serve, being more credible, dependable and more integrated in the services they provide, NGOs have a distinct edge over Government workers in convincing TB suspects to undergo diagnostic tests take their medicines regularly and report for the prescribed follow ups to ensure complete cure. TB can be cured and the epidemic reversed if governments accord it high priority, allocate adequate resources and provide strong administrative support for TB control. Tuberculosis is not merely a medical crisis. It is a major political crisis. It is a problem of developing countries where the world's poor largely live under adverse socio-economic conditions with limited access to health care. Stopping TB is a political decision determined by policy and decision makers who chart the course of a nation's future. TB cannot and will not be stopped unless those who want to stop it, enter into an open partnership with policy makers and planners to ensure that TB control programmes are not only built on sound public health principles but also with genuine concern for the millions of lives being needlessly lost every year, despite highly effective anti TB medicines and proven interventions.

The economic and social costs incurred by TB are particularly unnerving. In countries with already poor economies, this is even more devastating. Affecting people largely during their most productive years, leads to tremendous social, economic and psychological costs on families and societies and eventually on the growth of nations. The costs of "Inaction" leaves social scars. Families can lose 20-30% of annual household income when TB is left untreated. Inadequate TB treatment can lead to the development of multi-drug resistant TB. Multi-drug resistant TB is at least 100 times more expensive to cure. Policy makers have a big stake in stopping TB. The time has come for heads of state, finance and health ministers and other policy makers to provide the political leadership to reverse the uncontrollable spread of TB.

Total TB control costs have increased from about US $ 60 million in 2002 to a projected US$ 89 million in 2005; these figures may be overestimates because they assume that 75% of all DOT is undertaken at health facilities and that about 10,000 dedicated hospital beds are still being used for TB patients. In practice, community workers or volunteers may provide DOT to more than 25% of patients, at no cost to the health system, and increasing numbers of hospital beds previously dedicated to TB patients are being reallocated to other uses.

Government of India formulated and published schemes to promote participation of NGOs (2001) and private practitioners (2002) in implementing DOTS. During the past few years, several local initiatives have emerged in both urban and rural settings; the NTP has provided drugs free of charge and has taken responsibility for supervision and monitoring of laboratory and treatment services. The evaluated initiatives have shown an increase in case notification between 3% and 30%. Most projects have also achieved treatment success greater than the programme target of 85%. Encouraged by the success of these early experiments, the NTP, in collaboration with WHO, has embarked on scaling up PPM DOTS in 14 cities across the country. The strategy is to offer technical support to the city TB control programmes to facilitiate partnership developing through a fulltime PPM consultant assisted by two field supervisors. Future expansion of PPM DOTS will link all public, corporate, voluntary and private individual an institutional providers to the NTP. The programme has adapted the existing recording and reporting system in order to evaluate the PPM-DOTS activities. While progress has been made at the planned rate, actual expenditures were lower than budgets in both 2002 and 2003, so the cost of DOTS expansion has been lower than anticipated.

TB/HIV collaborative activities and initiatives to increase case detection and cure rates are not budgeted separately, and are thus included under other budget lines. Total TB control costs for 2002 and 2003 are based on expenditures, whereas those for 2004 and 2005 are based on budgets. Estimates of the costs of clinic visits and hospitalization are WHO estimates based on data provided by the NTP and from other sources.

Mobilizing all public sector health-care providers, especially medical colleges, as well as many private and other health-care providers outside the government service, is important to achieve swift progress, and successful efforts must continue to increase their involvement. Continuing human resource capacity building through revision of all training material should be a major planned activity. Maintaining quality during rapid growth is a priority, while addressing the urgent need for additional staff and laboratory support for the expanded services will be a major challenge in the coming years.

To address it, activities should include the development of guidelines for the management of paediatric TB and the introduction of a revised supervision and monitoring strategy with detailed indicators for activities at all levels. The most important constraint to the extension of quality TB services is the shortage of staff to manage the rapidly expanding programme, particularly at central and state levels. To improve this situation, additional technical staff should be recruited to assist the NTP manager, the limits on hiring contractual laboratory technicians can be relaxed and efforts should be made to achieve an adequate distribution of laboratory technicians to states where laboratories are understaffed. Sub-district contracted laboratory supervisors have greatly contributed to the success of the programme, and efforts should be made to sustain capacity over the next few years. Further political commitment at the state level is needed to ensure that the programme is fully staffed with stable management. The capacity of current staff can be increased through training programmes run in part by expert consultants. It is estimated that 3.4% of previously untreated TB cases are multi-drug resistant. Currently, the NTP does not supply second-line drugs for MDR-TB patients. There should be plans to build capacity at the state level for DRS and DOTS-Plus. Although MDR TB patients are not treated under the NTP, second-line drugs are widely available and used by many practitioners, both public and private.

During 2005, priority should be given to preparing the remaining districts for DOTS implementation. The preparatory activities include the improvement of laboratories and stores, recruitment, relocation and training of staff, and procurement of equipment and supplies. Some of the districts are in areas where operations are difficult to access and where intensive monitoring will be required. Diagnostic and laboratory services, TB/HIV coordination and links with other health-care providers and the community are three priority areas to improve programme performance. Joint HIV/TB coordination committees should be established at the national and state levels, and a referral system should be created at the subdistrict level between the existing NTP infrastructure and the VCT centres. Private and other health-care providers, including NGOs and medical colleges, play an extremely important role in India. Let us work together as one force to eradicate this ancient plague—TB, so that the last train to achieve the goal is not missed.

Chapter twenty-two

Paediatric Tuberculosis

Rennis Davis

INTRODUCTION

Tuberculosis remains one of the major diseases afflicting children throughout the world. Although the exact number of annual cases of childhood tuberculosis is unknown, WHO has estimated approximately 1.3 million new cases and 450,000 deaths per year in children due to tuberculosis.[1] Many of these cases go undiagnosed and untreated and many of these children could be salvaged if there were improvements in diagnosis and treatment available for children. It is difficult to confirm the diagnosis of tuberculosis by current microbiological methods. Even in industrialized countries the triad of a positive tuberculin skin test, radiographic and/or clinical manifestation consistent with tuberculosis and establishing recent link to a known infectious case of tuberculosis is the "gold standard" for diagnosis.

The natural history and clinical expression of infection due to mycobacterium tuberculosis differ substantially in children compared with adults. Tuberculosis is most common in young adults and children < 5 years of age. The age range of 5-14 years is often called the "favoured age" because in all human populations this group has the lowest rate of tuberculosis disease. Among adults, two third of cases occur in males, but there is no significant in gender distribution in childhood.

Tuberculosis in Children as Different from Tuberculosis in Adults

1. Children of different ages vary in terms of the risk of developing active tuberculosis and in the likelihood of transmission of infection.
2. Children rarely develop cavitary lesions.
3. Children more commonly have extra-pulmonary disease.
4. Children usually have smaller populations of M. tuberculosis organisms therefore, fewer children are culture positive and they have less secondary drug resistance.

5. Children respond to antituberculous medications differently: they tolerate higher relative doses per kilogram of body weight with fewer side effects.

Accurate diagnosis and effective treatment of tuberculosis disease and the identification of tuberculosis infection without disease, along with successful completion of preventive therapy are equally important for children as for adults. Children with tuberculosis respond well to and tolerate the same basic treatment regimens as used for adults.

BCG vaccination is routinely used throughout the world, but not in the United States. There is good evidence that BCG vaccination in children younger than 2 months of age protects children from miliary tuberculosis or tuberculosis meningitis, the data concerning the efficacy of various strains of BCG vaccination in preventing tuberculosis vary tremendously, with estimated protection reported as low as 0 percent as high as 80% in published studies.

Many experts in childhood tuberculosis feel that children have been neglected in the worldwide effort to control tuberculosis. There are many reasons for this including the fact that most children with tuberculosis are not infectious and therefore not considered to be as important as adults with contagious tuberculosis, the frustration at the difficulty in establishing a microbiological diagnosis of tuberculosis in children and the relative neglect of paediatricians and researchers in studying childhood tuberculosis. Infact there is rich scientific literature about childhood tuberculosis supporting simple practices, which if adequately put into place would greatly improve the ability to diagnose and treat children with tuberculosis.

EPIDEMIOLOGY

The actual global disease burden of childhood TB is not known but it has been assumed that 10% of the actual total TB case load is found amongst children. Global estimate of 1.3 million new cases and 4,50,000 deaths due to TB per year amongst children is reported. However these figures appear to be an underestimate of the size of the problem.

Proper identification and treatment of infectious cases will prevent childhood TB. However often childhood TB is accorded low priority by national TB control programs. Probable reasons include:

- Diagnostic difficulties.
- Rarely infectious.
- Limited resources.
- Controversy in effectiveness of BCG.
- Lack of data on treatment.[2]

However, this disregards the impact of tuberculosis on childhood morbidity and mortality. Pulmonary TB (PTB) to extrapulmonary TB (EPTB) ratio is usually around 3:1.[3] Good data on the burden of all forms of TB amongst children in India are not available. Most surveys conducted have focused on pulmonary TB and no significant population based studies on EPTB are available. Pulmonary TB is primarily an adult disease and it has been estimated that the 0-19-year-old population contains only 7% of the total prevalent cases.[3]

In general, pediatric tuberculosis case rates tend to mirror case rates in adults because children develop disease soon after acquiring the infection.

Risk for Progression to Tuberculosis Disease Once Infected

- Infants + children ≤ 4 years of age, especially those < 2 years of age.
- Adolescents and young adults.
- Persons co-infected with HIV.
- Persons with skin test conversion in the past 1-2 years.
- Persons who are immunocompromised especially in cases of malignancy and solid organ transplantation, immunosuppressive medical treatments, diabetes mellitus, chronic renal failure, silicosis and malnutrition.[4]

From a survey of RNTCP implemented districts in India, pediatric cases were seen to make up 3% of the total load of new cases registered under RNTCP. Lymph node TB cases predominated (>75%) amongst the pediatric EPTB cases registered under RNTCP. Many EPTB cases (>40% of LN cases) were diagnosed on clinical grounds with no confirmatory examinations performed. An almost equivalent number of pediatric TB cases being diagnosed in same health facilities, but were not being registered under RNTCP. Of those pediatric cases treated under RNTCP, cure and completion rates were both above 90%. Comparative figures for those cases not treated under RNTCP were 80% and 70% with default rates between 27-33%.[3]

The recent epidemic of HIV infection has had a profound affect on the epidemiology of tuberculosis among children because of two mechanisms:

1. HIV-infected adults with tuberculosis may transmit M. tuberculosis to children, some of whom will develop tuberculosis disease.
2. Children with HIV infection may be at increased risk of progressing from tuberculosis infection to disease.

Tuberculosis may be under diagnosed among HIV infected children because of its similarity in clinical presentation to other opportunistic infections common in acquired immunodeficiency syndrome (AIDS) and the difficulty confirming the diagnosis with positive cultures.

The incidence of drug-resistance tuberculosis has increased dramatically throughout the world. The major reasons for the development of drug resistance are poor patient adherence to treatment and provision of inadequate drug regimens by the physician or national tuberculosis program.

NATURAL HISTORY AND PATHOPHYSIOLOGY

Virtually all transmissions of mycobacterium tuberculosis from person to person are usually by airborne mucous droplets. Infectiousness is related to certain characteristics of person with tuberculosis and to specific environmental factors such as poor circulation of air. Factors that determine the risk of tuberculosis infection are the same for children and adults: the possibility of exposure to a person with active, infectious tuberculosis, the invectiveness and treatment status of the person with tuberculosis and the degree of exposure to the infectious individual. The more prolonged and closer the exposure to the infectious case, the greater the risk of infection. For children, this specifically includes exposure to caregivers with tuberculosis, such as relatives, neighbours, baby sitters, daycare providers, or teachers.[5] Poverty with resultant poor nutrition, overcrowded living conditions and inadequate medial care, continues to play a major role in the epidemiology of tuberculosis.

Children younger than 10 years of age are usually not considered to be contagious. There are several reasons for this: Children rarely have cavitary lesions, their pulmonary lesions generally have fewer numbers of M. tuberculosis organisms (therefore, they are more often culture negative), many children with tuberculosis have no or little cough and younger children are less capable of forcefully coughing and aerosolizing organisms in droplet nuclei.

The portal of entry for M. tuberculosis for almost all children is the respiratory tract. Ingestion of milk laden with bovine tuberculosis can lead to a gastrointestinal primary lesion. Rarely infection of the skin or mucous membrane can occur through an abrasion cut or insect bite.

The tubercle bacilli multiply initially within the alveoli and alveolar ducts. Some of the bacilli are ingested but not killed by macrophages that carry the organisms through lymphatic channels to the regional lymph nodes. The major groups of lymph node involved in children are in the hilar region, although paratracheal and subcranial nodes also may be involved, depending upon where the organisms lodge in the lung.

As with adults the incubation period between the time the tubercle bacilli are inhaled and the development of delayed hypersensitivity is usually between 3 and 12 weeks, most often 4 to 8 weeks. Some children experience a febrile illness that lasts from one to 3 weeks when hypersensitivity first develops. These children may have mild cough and other respiratory symptoms. The primary complex of tuberculosis consists of local reaction in the parenchyma of the lung where the organisms lodge and the inflammatory reaction of the associated lymph nodes. In most cases, the parenchymal portion of the primary complex heals completely by fibrosis and is of no clinical significance. Occasionally, the parenchymal lesion continues to enlarge resulting in focal pneumonitis and thickening of the overlying pleura. The foci in the regional lymph nodes develop some fibrosis but healing is usually less complete than in the parenchymal lesion. M. tuberculosis may persist for decades after fibrosis or calcification of the lymph nodes.[6]

Tuberculosis infection without the disease is the preclinical stage in which an individual has a positive tuberculin skin test but no signs or symptoms of disease and chest radiograph is normal. Tuberculosis represents clinical disease when the primary infection is not contained by the host response or when the latent infection reactivates, and clinical signs and symptoms are apparent. Estimates suggest that 5 to 10% of adults with M. tuberculosis infection progress to active disease at some time during their life.

Definition of a Positive Tuberculin Skin Test Reaction Result in Infants, Children and Adolescents

Indication > 5 mm

- Close contacts of known or suspected case of tuberculosis disease.
- Children having clinical or radiographic findings of tuberculosis disease.
- Children with immunosuppressive conditions, including HIV and organ transplantation.
- Patients receiving immunosuppressive therapy, including immunosuppressant doses of corticosteroids (≥ 15 mg/24 hr prednisone or equivalent for ≥ 1 month).

Induration ≥ 10 mm

- Infants and children ≤ 4 years of age.
- Children with underlying medical conditions or behaviours that increase risk (renal disease, hematological disorders, diabetes mellitus, malnutrition, injection drug use).
- Children with frequent exposure to adults at high risk.
- Birth or recent immigration (<5 years) from a high prevalence country.
- Children with travel to or exposure to visitors from high prevalence countries.

Induration ≥ 15 mm

- Children > 4 years of age and older without any risk factors.[4]

In some children, the lymph node becomes enlarged by the host inflammatory reaction. These lymph nodes then encroach on the regional bronchioles. Partial obstruction caused by external compression may lead at first to hyperinflation in the distal lung segment. This compression occasionally causes complete obstruction of the bronchus resulting in atelectasis of the lung segment. More often, inflamed caseous nodes attach to the bronchial wall and erode through it, leading to endobronchial tuberculosis and a fistulous tract. The extrusion of infected caseous material into the bronchus transmits infection to the lung parenchyma causing bronchial obstruction and further atelectasis. The resulting lesion, which is a combination of the pneumonitis and atelectasis, is often referred to as a collapse consolidation or segmental lesion. If the subcranial nodes are involved the enlargement may cause invasion of adjacent structures such as the pericardium or esophagus, resulting in pericarditis or a tracheoesophageal fistula, respectively.

During the development of the parenchymal and lymph node lesions, tubercle bacilli from the primary complex spread via the blood stream and lymphatics to many parts of the body. Sites that are most commonly seeded are the apices of the lungs, liver, spleen, meninges, peritoneum, lymph nodes, pleura and bone. The dissemination can involve either large numbers of bacilli, which leads to disseminated tuberculosis or small numbers of bacilli that create microscopic tuberculosis foci scattered in the tissues. Initially, these metastatic foci are clinically inapparent but they can be the origin of both extrapulmonary tuberculosis and reactivation pulmonary tuberculosis in later life.

Massive lymphohematogenous dissemination leading to miliary or disseminated disease occurs in only 0.5 to 2% of infected children but occurs early after the initial infection. Clinically significant lymph node or lung tuberculosis usually appears within 3 to 9 months. However, lesions in bones and joints and kidneys take much longer to develop, often several years after the infection first occur. In summary, vast majority of cases of tuberculosis in children occur within 1 year of the infection meaning that tuberculosis disease in a child is a marker of recent transmission of the organism.[6]

CLINICAL, RADIOGRAPHIC AND LABORATORY FINDINGS

The majority of children with tuberculosis infection develop neither signs nor symptoms at any time. Occasionally the initiation of the infection is marked by several days of low-grade fever and mild cough. Rarely, the child experiences a clinically significant disease with high fever, cough, malaise and flu like symptoms that resolve within a week. Most children who develop tuberculosis disease experience pulmonary manifestations, but approx. 25 to 35 percent of children have an extra pulmonary presentation. The most common extra pulmonary form of tuberculosis is lymphatic disease accounting for about two thirds of cases of extra pulmonary tuberculosis. However, the second most common form is meningeal disease occurring in 13% of patients.[6]

Pulmonary Disease

Depending on its progression, active pulmonary tuberculosis in children manifests in a variety of forms including:

- Endobronchial disease with focal lymphadenopathy.
- Progressive pulmonary disease.
- Pleural involvement, and
- Reactivated pulmonary disease.

The most common form is endobronchial disease with focal lymphadenopathy resulting from spread of the tubercle bacillus from the alveoli to both the bronchioles and lymphatic. Subsequent drainage to the lymph nodes along with the host response of activated macrophage and delayed hypersensitivity, leads to a significant inflammatory response and lymph node enlargement. Lymph node enlargement can impinge on proximal anatomical sites and result in various clinical manifestations such as bronchial obstruction, odynophagia with esophageal compression and vocal cord or hemidiaphragmatic paralysis caused by local nerve compression. Bronchial obstruction can lead to a "collapse consolidation" picture on chest roentgenogram, usually with minimal symptoms or signs suggestive of foreign-body aspiration or just a persistent cough.

Progressive primary pulmonary tuberculosis results when the focal lesion progresses to a large caseous mass. The caseous mass often drains into proximal bronchi and cavitates. This form of pulmonary disease is rare in children but occurs more commonly in young infants or persons with abnormal cell-mediated immunity. These young children often appear very ill, with marked weight loss, fever and cough. Classic signs of pneumonia are often evident over the progressive lesions: dullness to percussion egophony, decreased breath sounds, and rales.

Pleural involvement in primary pulmonary tuberculosis is generally uncommon, occurring more often in older children or adolescents. Clinical presentation is one of pneumonia with a pleural effusion and persistent fever. Mediastinal shift along with marked shortness of breath and tachypnoea can occur with large effusions.

Reactivation tuberculosis occurs primarily in older children and adolescents. It is the result of activation of an old, latent focus of M tuberculosis infection spread to that site lymphohematogenously. Generally, this is a focal process, limited by previous host response and sensitivity to M. tuberculosis such that the reactivated infection undergoes caseation and liquefaction. The clinical presentation is usually subacute with weight loss, fatigue, fever, cough and (rarely) hemoptysis.[7]

Extrapulmonary Tuberculosis

Extrapulmonary tuberculosis commonly includes:

- Peripheral lymphadenopathy in approx. 60% of patients.
- Tuberculous meningitis (10-15%).
- Infection of bones or joints (5%), and
- Miliary tuberculosis (infection at several distant sites) in 5% of patients.

Peripheral tuberculous lymphadenitis generally is the result of local spread from the primary site of infection, especially to supraclavicular or paratracheal nodes. Lymphohematogenous dissemination can spread infection to distant lymph nodes from the primary infection. Rarely peripheral adenitis is the result of a primary extrapulmonary site of infection. Tuberculous lymphadenitis usually presents as enlarged, firm, nontender lymph nodes with little erythema or fluctuance. Weight loss, fatigue, malaise, or fever is either absent or minimal. The adenitis can progress to caseation and necrosis and cause erythema, fluctuance and occasionally spontaneous drainage. The lymph nodes most commonly involved are the anterior or posterior cervical and supraclavicular lymph nodes. Often a biopsy and culture are necessary to distinguish other common causes of lymphadenitis and tuberculous or nontuberculous mycobacterial lymphadenitis.[8]

Tuberculous meningitis is the most common cause of death from tuberculosis because of the delay that usually occurs in making the diagnosis. It occurs most commonly in children less than 6 years of age. Lymphohematogenous spread seeds foci in the brain, meninges or both and caseation can lead to extension into the subarachnoid space. Hydrocephalus occurs if there is obstruction of CSF flow. Extension to the basilar meninges can cause compression of the third, sixth and seventh nerves, resulting in paresis, paralysis, or both. The clinical picture of tuberculosis meningitis is insidious and requires a high index of suspicion to make a timely diagnosis. Initially nonspecific signs and symptoms (fever, vomiting, decreased appetite, and behavioural changes) predominate. After 1 to 2 weeks, focal signs are evident, including vomiting stiff neck, altered sensorium, or seizures. Altered deep tendon reflexes, cranial nerve palsies or unintelligible speech may appear. The illness can progress to severe cerebral damage despite early diagnosis and intervention, causing decerebrate or decorticate positioning, opisthotonos, deteriorating mental status, coma and death.

Miliary tuberculosis is caused by the rupture of caseous material into a blood vessel, resulting in hematogenous spread to numerous sites throughout the body. Like tuberculosis meningitis miliary tuberculosis is a complication of primary tuberculosis in young children. Approximately one-third of children with miliary tuberculosis present with meningitis as one of the many involved sites. The presentation of miliary tuberculosis depends on the specific sites involved. It can occur either subacutely with weight loss, fatigue malaise and low-grade fever or acutely with high fever and rapid onset of associated symptoms. The child usually has lymphadenopathy, hepatosplenomegaly and a paucity of respiratory signs. Respiratory manifestations often evolve and include cough, tachypnoea, cyanosis and respiratory distress. Subtle findings such as papular, necrotic or purpuric lesion on the skin or choroidal tubercles on the retina should be carefully sought in the physical examination.

Skeletal tuberculosis is a late complication of lymphohematogenous spread of bacilli usually presenting years after the primary infection. Infants and young children are at greater risk of tuberculosis of the bone or joints because of the increased likelihood of lymphohematogenous dissemination and increased vascularity of their bones during growth. The focal infection often begins in the metaphysis from bacilli seeding the endarteries. Endarteritis leads to local bony destruction and subsequent drainage into the adjacent joint capsule or through a sinus tract to the skin. The most common sites involved are the large weight bearing bones or joints such as the vertebrae (30-40%), hip (7%), knee (7%) and elbow (5%). Tuberculosis of bone or joint presents either acutely or subacutely, as do the other common pyogenic bacterial skeletal infections. Vertebral tuberculosis may be very insidious, presenting with signs or referred pain, abnormal posturing or even a paravertebral abscess. Bony destruction with bone deformity is a late sign of skeletal tuberculosis.[7]

Other rarer forms of **extrapulmonary tuberculosis** include sites such as the middle ear or mastoid, kidneys, pericardium, eyes, skin, abdominal and gastrointestinal, or genitourinary. A comprehensive description of each one of them is beyond the scope of this article.

Tuberculosis in Newborn Infant

Can occur either as:

- Congenital tuberculosis, or
- From postnatally acquired infection.

Congenital tuberculosis occurs rarely. Infection of the fetus can occur through transplacental spread of bacilli through the umbilical vein, bacilli reaching the amniotic fluid from tuberculous endometritis placentitis or both or from ingestion of infected amniotic fluid at the time of delivery. The clinical presentation of congenital tuberculosis commonly begins in the second or third week of life and is similar to that of bacterial sepsis or other congenital infections. Signs and symptoms often include poor feeding and poor weight gain, jaundice hepatosplenomegaly, abdominal distension, cough, tachypnoea, irritability, lethargy and lymphadenopathy. Diagnostic criteria for congenital tuberculosis require the illness to have begun in the first weeks of the infants life, the mother to have documented tuberculosis and the infant to have a positive culture for M. tuberculosis or preferably, histological evidence of caseating granuloma or a primary hepatic complex.

Perinatal tuberculosis is more common than congenital tuberculosis but has a lower mortality rate. Clinical presentation is usually delayed until the patient is 1 to 3 months of age and varies according to the infecting dose of bacilli and the sites involved. The clinical presentation may suggest congenital tuberculosis, tuberculous meningitis, miliary tuberculosis or primary pulmonary tuberculosis. Diagnosis of active tuberculosis in the mother or other close contact of the infant is essential, particularly in documenting postnatal transmission.[9]

LABORATORY EVALUATION

General laboratory test such as a complete blood count and differential cell counts are usually normal in children with tuberculosis. When pleural tuberculosis is present, pleural fluid is usually yellow and occasionally tinged with blood. The chemistry results are indicative of a mild exudate; specific gravity is usually 1.012 to 1.025, the protein level is usually 2 to 4 q/dl and the glucose may be low normal range (20-40 mg/dl). Most typically, there are several hundred to several thousand white blood cells/mm^3 with an early predominance of polymorphonuclear cells followed by a high proportion of lymphocyte. Acid-fast smear of the fluid are usually negative because of the relative paucity of organisms. Cultures are positive in only 30 to 70% of cases. Biopsy of the pleura is more likely to yield a positive acid-fast stain or culture and evidence of granuloma formation can be demonstrated.

In cases of tuberculous meningitis, the CSF leukocyte count usually ranges from 10 to 500 cells/mm^3 but occasionally is higher. Lymphocytes usually predominate but there may be more leukocytes initially. The CSF glucose level is typically < 40 mg/dl but rarely goes below 20 mg/dl. The protein level is elevated and may be markedly high (400-5000 mg/dl) secondary to hydrocephalus and spinal block. The success of microscopic examinations of an acid-fast stain of CSF and myobacterial culture is directly related to the amount of CSF sampled. When 5 to 10 ml of lumbar CSF is obtained, the acid-fast stain of the CSF sediment is positive in upto 30% of case and the culture is positive in 70%.

The most important laboratory test for the diagnosis and management of tuberculosis in adults is the acid-fast stain and culture of sputum. The best culture specimen for pulmonary tuberculosis in the child is the early morning gastric aspirate obtained before the child has arisen and peristalsis has emptied the stomach of the pooled secretions that have been swallowed overnight. Unfortunately, even under optimum conditions, three gastric aspirates yield M. tuberculosis in < 50% of cases, negative cultures never exclude the diagnosis of tuberculosis in a child. The yield from flexible bronchoscopy is less than from properly obtained gastric aspirates. Unfortunately, the acid-fast stain of either sputum or gastric contents in small children is positive in < 10% cases. Bronchial secretion obtained by stimulating cough with an aerosol solution can be used for culture in older children.

Fortunately, the need for culture confirmation is usually low. If the child has a positive tuberculin skin test, clinical or radiographic findings suggestive of tuberculosis and known contact with an adult case of tuberculosis, the child should be treated for tuberculosis disease. The drug susceptibility test (DST) results from the adult case can be used to determine the best therapeutic regimen for the child. Although the polymerase chain reaction (PCR) to amplify DNA sequences specific for M. tuberculosis has been applied to children, the yield is not much greater than from culture and the specificity is low enough that false positive result do occur. In general, PCR may be an aid in the diagnosis of extrapulmonary tuberculosis.[6]

TREATMENT

To seek consensus on improved case detection and improved treatment outcomes for all diagnosed paediatric TB cases in India, a workshop was held in New Delhi on 6th and 7th August 2003. Following guidelines were formulated for diagnosis and treatment of paediatric TB cases under RNTCP[2]:

1. Diagnosis

Suspect cases of PTB will include children presenting with fever and/or cough for more than 3 weeks, with or without weight loss or no weight gain and history of contact with a suspected or diagnosed case of active TB disease within the last 2 years. Diagnosis to be based on a combination of clinical presentation, sputum examination, wherever possible, chest X-ray (PA view), Mantaux test (1 TU PPD RT 23 with Tween 80, positive if induration > 10 mm after 48-72 hours) and history of contact. A medical officer should make diagnosis of TB in children. Where diagnostic difficulties are faced referral of the child should be made to a paediatrician for further management. The existing RNTCP case definitions will be used for all cases diagnosed.

2. Treatment of Paediatric TB

DOTS is the recommended strategy for treatment of TB and all paediatric TB patients should be registered under RNTCP. Intermittent short course chemotherapy given under direct observation, as advocated in the RNTCP, should be used in children.

Table 22.1: RNTCP treatment regimens[10]

Category of treatment	*Type of patients*	*TB treatment regimens*	
		Intensive phase	*Continuation phase*
CAT I	• New sputum smear positive PTB • Seriously ill* sputum smear negative PTB • Seriously ill extra pulmonary TB	*** $2H_3R_3Z_3E_3$	$4H_3R_3$
CAT II	• Sputum smear positive relapse • Sputum smear positive treatment failure	$2S_3H_3R_3Z_3E_3$/ $1H_3R_3Z_3E_3$	$5H_3R_3E_3$
CAT III	• Sputum smear negative • Extrapulmonary TB, not seriously ill**	$2H_3R_3Z_3$	$4H_3R_3$

* Seriously ill sputum smear-negative PTB includes all forms of PTB other than primary complex; seriously ill EPTB includes TB meningitis (TBM), disseminated/miliary TB, TB pericarditis TB peritonitis and intestinal TB, bilateral or extensive pleurisy, spinal TB with or without neurological complications, genitourinary tract TB, bone and joint TB.

** Not seriously ill EPTB includes lymph node TB and unilateral pleural effusion.

*** Prefix indicates month and subscript indicates thrice weekly.

In patients with TBM on category I treatment, the four drugs used during the intensive phase should be HRZS or HRZE. Continuation phase of treatment in TBM and spinal TB with neurological complication should be given for 6-7 months, extending the total duration of treatment to 8-9 months.

Steroids should be used initially in hospitalized cases of TBM and TB pericarditis and reduced gradually over 6-8 weeks.

In all instances before starting a child on category II treatment, a paediatrician or TB expert should examine him, wherever available. As recommended by WHO and in view of the growing evidence that the use of ethambutol in young children is safe. Ethambutol is to be used as per RNTCP regimen for all age groups.[11]

To assist in calculating required dosages and administration of anti-TB drugs for children, the medication should be made available in the form of combipacks in patient-wise boxes, linked to the child's weight.

3. Chemoprophylaxis

Asymptomatic children under 6 years of age, exposed to an adult with infections (smear, positive) tuberculosis, from the same household, will be given 6 months of isoniazid (5 mg per kg daily) chemoprophylaxis.

4. Monitoring and Evaluation

Paediatric focused monitoring may preferably be an integral part of the program. Wherever possible, follow up sputum examination is to be performed with the same frequency as in adults. Clinical or symptomatic improvement is to be assessed at the end of the intensive phase of treatment and at the end of treatment. Improvement should be judged by absence of fever or cough, a decrease in the size of lymph nodes, weight gain. Radiological improvement is to be assessed by chest X-ray examination in all smear negative pulmonary TB cases at the end of treatment.[2]

PREVENTION

There are numerous methods of preventing the spread of tuberculosis, such as effective treatment of active, infections of pulmonary tuberculosis, chemoprophylaxis, environmental controls (masks, adequate ventilation, ultraviolet lighting and isolation), contact or associate investigation; and vaccination with BCG. Methods that are particularly important in paediatrics include prophylactic isoniazid for high-risk contacts of a patient with contagious tuberculosis, preventive isoniazid in a person with tuberculin conversion (to prevent the development of tuberculosis disease), and BCG vaccination in areas with a high prevalence of tuberculosis.

Prophylactic Therapy

An infant or child (< 6 years) who is exposed to a case of active pulmonary tuberculosis and whose initial tuberculosis skin test is negative should receive isoniazid for 6 months in an attempt to prevent infection. Renewed efforts to treat active tuberculosis effectively in the adult must be undertaken at the same time to decrease the risk of transmission.

BCG Vaccination

In much of the world, the only method available to prevent tuberculosis in children is administration of a Bacilli Calmette-Guerin (BCG) vaccine. When considering the total body of literature of BCG vaccination of children, the general conclusion is that the BCG vaccines prevent 60 to 90% of serious tuberculosis cases in children. Clearly, the BCG vaccines are better than no method of prevention, but they are not capable of completely preventing tuberculosis disease in a population of children. The presence of HIV infection in the child is an absolute contraindication to giving BCG vaccine, but internationally, the presence of asymptomatic HIV infection is not considered a contraindication to BCG vaccination.

Contact Investigation

Contact investigation and associate investigation are essential components of any program of tuberculosis prevention.[12] A contact investigation is the systematic evaluation of the tuberculosis status of the contacts of an identified case of active tuberculosis. An associate investigation examines the tuberculosis status of all close contacts of a child with a positive tuberculin skin test to identify the source case and other infected contacts. Several investigations have shown that when contact investigations are not conducted well or completely, preventable cases of tuberculosis in children inevitably occur.

REFERENCES

1. Kochi, A. The global tuberculosis situation and the new control strategy of World Health Organization. *Tubercle* 1991;71:1-6.
2. Chauhan LS, Arora VK Management of Pediatric Tuberculosis under the Revised National Tuberculosis Control Programme. *Indian J. Pediatrics* 2004;71:341-343.
3. Central TB division (CTD), DGHS, MoHFW, Government of India. TB India 2003: *TNTCP status report Delhi CTD:*2003.
4. Behrman, Kliegman, Jenson. *Nelson Textbook of Pediatrics*. Mycobacterial infections. 17th Edition. Elsevier Publishers, Indian Reprint 2004;958-975.
5. Leggiadro,. RJ, Callory, B, Dowdy, S, *et al*. An outbreak of tuberculosis in a family day care home. *Paediatr Infect Dis J* 1989;8:52-54.
6. Jeffrey, R, Starke, Tuberculosis in children. *Semin. Respir Crit Care Med* 2004;25(3):353-364.
7. William, N., Rom, Stuart M, Garay. Tuberculosis; *Tuberculosis in children.* First Edition. Little, Brown and Company 1996;675-688.
8. Wier, MR, Thornton, GF. Extrapulmonary tuberculosis: Experiences of a community hospital and review of the literature. *Am J Med* 1985;79:467-478.

9. Nemir RL, O'Hare, D. Congenital tuberculosis: Review and diagnostic guidelines. *Am J Dis Child* 1985;139:284-287.
10. World Health Organization. WHO. Treatment of tuberculosis. Guidelines for National Programs. Geneva WHO; 2003 (*WHO/CDS/TB* 2003:313).
11. Graham, S.M., Daley, HM, Banerjee A, Salani Pani, FM, Harries, AD. Ethambutol in tuberculosis: time to reconsider? *Arch Dis Child* 1998;79:274-278.
12. American Thoracic Society, Control of tuberculosis in the United States. *Am Rev Respir Dis* 1992;146(6):1623-1633.

Index